Challenges in Midwifery Care

======= RELATED TITLES FROM MACMILLAN =======

Sheila C. Hunt and Anthea Symonds
The Social Meaning of Midwifery
ISBN 0–333–60877–1

Anthea Symonds and Sheila C. Hunt
The Midwife and Society
ISBN 0–333–63038–6

Rosamund Bryar
Theory for Midwifery Practice
ISBN 0–333–58867–3

Challenges in Midwifery Care

Edited by

ISHBEL KARGAR

and

SHEILA C. HUNT

MACMILLAN

First published 1997 by
MACMILLAN PRESS LTD
Houndmills, Basingstoke, Hampshire RG21 6XS
and London
Companies and representatives
throughout the world

ISBN 0–333–60904–2 paperback

A catalogue record for this book is available
from the British Library.

This book is printed on paper suitable for recycling and
made from fully managed and sustained forest sources.

10   9   8   7   6   5   4   3   2   1
06   05   04   03   02   01   00   99   98   97

Editing and origination by
Aardvark Editorial, Mendham, Suffolk

Printed in Hong Kong

CONTENTS

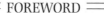

This book emerged from the experiences of midwives as they met together at regional meetings of the Association of Radical Midwives. It is clear that in that supportive environment they thought, felt, listened, reflected and learned more about the practice of midwifery. The ideas were sometimes new, sometimes different, and often about unusual experiences.

In this text are ideas, rich sources of information, references and those 'tricks of the trade' that are often difficult or impossible to locate in standard textbooks.

For midwives who are passionate about their practice and intent on improving the childbirth experience for women, this book is a gem. It will be invaluable for midwives seeking advice and sometimes inspiration on giving care to special people in special circumstances. I commend this book to midwives everywhere.

Caroline Flint
London, 1996

ACKNOWLEDGEMENTS

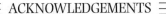

The editors would like to thank the sterling efforts made by the contributors in bringing the chapters in this book to publication. In addition, we would like to thank Kerry Lawrence for believing in the ideas, and Carrie Walker for her patience, guidance and perseverance.

Rachel Celia RGN, RM, DipCoun, MSc is a freelance psychotherapist and consultant. She was Clinical Nurse Specialist (Haemoglobinopathies), West Lambeth CCT for 11 years and is currently setting up a specialist counselling agency to meet the needs of people affected by serious childhood illness.

Mandy Churcher RN, RM, ADM, PGCEA, MEd is a midwife teacher at the City University, St Bartholomew's School of Nursing and Midwifery. As well as the care of pregnant travellers, her research interests include the history of midwifery practice and education.

Karen Connolly RGN, RM, DPSM is a maternity ward team leader at St Mary's Hospital, Manchester. Her interest in supporting the parents of babies with a congenital abnormality, and her awareness of the crucial role of communication skills, were inspired by the birth of her daughter in 1987.

Jean Davies RN RM MSc is a Regional Officer with the Royal College of Midwives. She initiated the Newcastle Community Midwifery Care Project for which she received a *Nursing Times* 3M award and a Brenda Mee memorial prize. She worked as a midwife in an inner city for ten years, then as a research midwife for the Northern Region Home Birth study before joining the RCM.

Joanna Hindley BA, RM is a staff midwife at the Birmingham Women's Hospital and an independent midwife practising in the Birmingham area. Her interest in female genital mutilation stems from research she undertook for her first degree and her previous employment with the Quakers at the United Nations in Geneva where she promoted awareness of FGM as a human rights issue.

Sheila C. Hunt MSc Econ, MBA, RGN, RM, PGCE is Professor of Midwifery for the Birmingham Women's Health Care NHS Trust and the Head of the School of Women's Health Studies at the University of Central England in Birmingham. She is the author, with Anthea Symonds, of *The Social Meaning of Midwifery* and *The Midwife and Society*.

Ishbel Kargar SRN, SCM came back to midwifery on her return to the UK in 1981 after living in Iran for 25 years. Joining the Association of Radical Midwives gave her much appreciated support at this time and she has been Administrative Secretary since 1983. Ishbel retired from clinical midwifery practice in 1992 and has spent two years as a *Nursing Times* Arena columnist.

Jennifer Kelsall MSc, RGN, RM, MTD is Core Midwife (Delivery Suite) at South Manchester University Hospitals NHS Trust. In 1992 Jennifer won a *Nursing Times* 3M Award for her Maternity Care for the Deaf project. She is an RCM Representative on the Maternity Alliance Disability Working Group.

Jenny Kitzinger BA, MA is Senior Research Fellow in the Mass Media Research Unit, Department of Sociology at Glasgow University. Jenny's previous experience includes voluntary work at a centre for incest survivors and research into media representation of sexual violence against children, maternity service provision, and public understanding of AIDS. She is co-author of *Great Expectations: A prospective study of women's expectations and experience of childbirth* (Books for Midwives Press, 1997).

Pippa MacKeith RN, RM, BSc is a specialist midwife with a community team for homeless people, Nottingham Community Health (NHS) Trust. Pippa has over 17 years experience of practical midwifery, five of which were spent at 45 Cope Street, Nottingham running groups for young mothers.

Sarah Montagu MA, RGN, DPSN, RM is a team midwife at the City Hospital, Birmingham. Prior to her midwifery training, Sarah studied Hebrew at Cambridge University and was subsequently involved in inter-faith work between Jews, Muslims and Christians. This experience has given her a particular interest in issues relating to childbirth in different cultures.

Rosemary Phillipson RN, RM, HV, CertHealthEd is a health promotion group worker working with young women at 45 Cope Street, Nottingham. Rosemary trained as a midwife at St Mary's Hospital, Manchester, and subsequently spent six years as a community midwife in Staffordshire.

Mary Sidebotham RN, RM, DPSM/ADM is a clinical midwife at St Mary's Hospital, Manchester. She is also Donor Recruitment Coordinator for NEEDS (the National Egg and Embryo Donation Society). Mary is studying for an MA in health care, ethics and the law and her thesis subject is egg donation.

Catherine Siney SRN, RM is a specialist midwife (drug liaison) at Liverpool Women's Hospital. Catherine was involved in the setting up of maternity and gynaecology services and advice for women who were drug users, are alcoholics or who are HIV or hepatitis positive.

Meg Taylor BSc, MSc, RM, DipCouns, BAC Accredited is a counsellor in private practice. After being diagnosed with MS in 1985, Meg had two children (both born at home) and has a special interest in the emotional aspects of childbearing.

This book is dedicated to those special women and their families from whom we have learned so much and who need from midwives that extra special care in childbirth.

One of the guiding principles of the Association of Radical Midwives when planning its quarterly meetings around the UK is that speakers and skill-sharing workshop leaders can usually be recruited from local midwives. Those doubting this, feeling that 'experts' from elsewhere would have been better, have often been pleasantly surprised that a really informative, instructive, interesting and stimulating day has been enjoyed by everyone, listening and learning from local colleagues with hidden talents.

This book is a demonstration of this principle and proof of the valuable knowledge and experience possessed by 'ordinary' midwives who have accepted the challenge presented by a particular aspect of their practice. They have all seen that some women in their care have special needs, over and above the usual maternity care, that must be met. These colleagues of ours made it their business to learn more about the particular difficulties of such women and have, in the process, built up an impressive body of practical expertise and theoretical knowledge, which they now share with us.

Many midwives will read the contents page and comment that they are already dealing with such 'special' circumstances quite adequately. We have no doubt that this is so, and would hope that such is the case for the majority of practitioners. Nevertheless, midwives will surely agree that they can never stop learning, and if the special situations dealt with in these chapters highlight aspects of care that have not previously been addressed, the book will have served its purpose in challenging midwives to enhance the care they provide.

Some of the problems dealt with are less common, and midwives may be forgiven for reading these chapters with only professional curiosity, rather than as examples of situations they may have to deal with themselves. However, midwifery is continually widening its knowledge base, and just as we learned about Bandl's ring, probably never actually to see one, we also need to learn how to help a woman whose needs may be out of the ordinary, but who may be the next client in our practice.

The book is aimed at midwives in clinical practice caring for women with special needs, for whom the usual approach to maternity care has to be modified.

Until comparatively recently, good midwifery texts were few in number, and although one or two of these have almost attained the status of a 'bible' of midwifery knowledge, they contained only passing reference to a few special needs in pregnancy and childbirth, such as some physical handicaps, and specific medical or social conditions presenting an element of risk to the pregnancy or to the woman. None of these has so far addressed in any depth the requirements of particular groups of women, or offered substantial assistance to midwives caring for these women by way of information about support groups, extensive reference texts and help on a more practical level.

This situation is now changing, as midwives develop the skills and discover the joys and rewards of research, often inspired by problems encountered in their own clinical practice. Such studies are welcomed by their colleagues, not least because the situations dealt with often reflect their own practice and are therefore highly relevant.

There is a growing recognition that there is no single 'best' system of maternity care for all women, and that not only individual women, but also certain *groups* of women, have special needs. The contributors to this book realise that while addressing the problems of particular 'groups', there must always be an awareness that the women concerned are first and foremost individuals, with their own needs and desires, albeit having many of those needs in common with other women with similar difficulties.

The authors examine these needs with particular reference to midwifery care, and in exploring the problems try to offer a deeper understanding than has hitherto been available to those seeking it. It is acknowledged that almost all of these 'special needs' groups have already been identified within society, and some suggestions for improving their maternity care have been made, either in passing while discussing other problems, perhaps in a textbook, in research study, in occasional professional journals or in the information leaflets produced by campaigning and self-help groups. This book gathers a significant amount of this scattered but valuable information, plus additional material, into one text which we hope will become a book of choice for midwives wishing to learn more about special needs.

Most of the chapters have been written by practising midwives in their spare time, drawing on their own experiences and clinical practice, using case studies where possible to illustrate their work. One author is not a midwife but has made a valuable contribution to the book, which will be welcomed by midwives encountering the problems she deals with. Some of the writers are putting pen to paper for the first time, having been encouraged to make their work more widely known, often after speaking at a local meeting.

The final chapter considers a relatively new challenge, faced by all midwives – the challenge of change in the organisation and philosophy of midwifery as a result of 'Changing Childbirth' and other documents. This chapter analyses the origins of change and explores key management theories. It considers why individuals and organisations resist change and looks at strategies for 'coping with it'. It seeks to support and understand midwives as they support and understand women during a period of unprecedented 'upheaval'.

Throughout the book, the authors' deep understanding of the feelings, frustrations, emotions and needs of childbearing women is evident, encouraging fellow midwives to accept the challenge, to practise through listening to the women in their care with patience and empathy, and really to be 'with woman'. Only thus will midwifery move forward to the woman-centred, sympathetic service that is becoming recognised as the only right way to practise.

We are very proud to have been associated with these people and shall be eternally grateful for the opportunity of helping them to bring their special experiences, studies and findings to the attention of an even wider audience.

Ishbel Kargar
Sheila Hunt
January 1997

CHAPTER ONE

Haemoglobinopathies and pregnancy

Rachel Celia

Haemoglobinopathies (HbOs), including sickle cell disease and thalassaemia, are inherited abnormalities of haemoglobin manufacture. They can occur in people of all races and origins, although they are more common in people who have non-northern European ancestry. All women at risk of having inherited an HbO should be offered antenatal testing, and appropriate laboratory and counselling services must be provided to enable them to make informed choices.

Sickle cell disease has an effect not only on the bodily structures of the individual, but also on every aspect of that person's life. She comes to her pregnancy not only with particular health needs, but also with complicated psychological needs. Childbearing has additional risks for both the mother and the baby, and the mother should be cared for by experienced obstetricians and haematologists.

The midwife's role is crucial, however, in providing a responsive and appropriate environment. The challenge to her as a professional is to facilitate a situation within which the woman's complex and changing needs can be determined, respected and met. In order to achieve this, and to empower her client, the midwife will need to use all her skills of communication and observation:

> These are special patients needing special care... for optimum results what is needed are eyes trained to see, ears trained to hear, hands trained to feel, a mind trained to monitor, interpret and act, and a kind heart. (Klufio *et al.* 1977, quoted by Konotey-Ahulu 1991)

A successful response to the midwifery challenge will provide the best possible opportunity for a healthy mother and baby to form the essential relationship base they need in order to support them through the many difficult times that they are likely to have to deal with in their life together.

A basic knowledge of the physiology of blood formation will be useful in understanding this topic. For more information, see the Further Reading list at the end of this chapter.

4

WHAT ARE HAEMOGLOBINOPATHIES?

Sickle haemoglobin (HbS) is one of several hundred inherited abnormalities of haemoglobin (Hb) manufacture collectively called 'haemoglobinopathies', which are mostly just different forms of the common adult Hb (HbA). HbOs are determined by recessive genes, so do not usually manifest themselves as symptomatic illnesses unless they are inherited from both parents. They are not sex linked, although it has been suggested that sickle cell diseases may affect males and females slightly differently (Leavel & Ford 1983).

People who have inherited the HbS gene from only one parent are said to have sickle cell trait (HbAS) or to be carriers. Such people are symptom free because their HbA protects them. It is similarly possible for a person to have a trait of any of the other HbOs.

There are two kinds of HbO. One affects the structure of the Hb molecule, and this group includes HbS and HbC which is another common HbO. The other kind affects the amounts made of the component parts of the Hb molecule; this group includes the thalassaemias.

HbOs can be inherited in any combination. HbS, for example, can be inherited in combination with HbS, HbC or beta thalassaemia. This results in the conditions sickle cell anaemia (HbSS), HbS/HbC disorder and sickle/beta thalassaemia (HbS/B thal) respectively. The expression of these disorders can vary from person to person, and from one period of life to another for the same individual. HbSS and one form of HbS/B thal generally, but not always, cause the most clinically serious problems.

The many different HbOs are generally believed to be associated with people from different parts of the world. It is important to remember when providing health care that most HbOs are much more widely distributed than is commonly believed, and that those at risk can certainly not be identified by visual appearance. HbS, for example, is just as common in parts of Greece as it is in parts of Nigeria.

SICKLE CELL DISEASE

In HbS, the genetic mutation causes an amino acid substitution in the beta-globin chains of the Hb. This changes the solubility of the Hb when it is deoxygenated, resulting in the formation of polymer chains, which deform the cells from within. This in turn causes the characteristic sickle-shaped cells after which the condition is named, which can become lodged in the capillaries, causing vaso-occlusion.

As deoxygenation of the Hb is a major factor in sickle cell disease, anything which increases oxygen requirements is a risk. So too are dehydration, changes in the pH of the blood, infection, fever and extremes of, or sudden changes in, temperature.

The vaso-occlusive episodes may occur at any time and at any site in the body, where they cause excruciating pain and progressive deterioration of body structures. The pain may be of such severity for people to believe that the pain will kill them. These painful crises are therefore not only experienced as torture, but also as life-threatening or even near-death experiences. This has a profound effect on the person. The acute episodes, or 'crises', are identified by the nature of the individual episode. For example, if pain is the presenting problem, it is called a 'painful crisis'; if the lungs or chest are involved, it is called a 'chest crisis'. These crises can be life-threatening and can cause intense fear and anxiety. Body organs (some of them vital) will be progressively damaged, resulting in further health problems.

The deformed red cells have a greatly reduced lifespan (10–14 days), resulting in a profound lifelong haemolytic anaemia. People with HbSS usually have an Hb level of 7–9 g/dl. However, the lifelong nature of this state results in an adaptive process that allows the more efficient utilisation of the available Hb. Maternal anaemia can never be taken lightly, however, and requires diligent monitoring during pregnancy.

In addition to these effects, many other medical emergencies may arise, and sufferers are particularly susceptible to overwhelming infection. Sudden and/or early death may occur at any time.

Reports regarding mortality rates vary. In infancy, they are as high as 30 per cent in some studies (Horn *et al.* 1986). Throughout childhood, the mortality rate falls, only to rise again steeply in the mid-thirties.

When well, people with sickle cell disorders are said to be in 'steady state'. Apart from penicillin prophylaxis for children under 16 and folic acid (to facilitate red cell production), treatment is unlikely to be necessary. Treatment during a crisis is symptomatic (analgesia, antibiotics, rehydration and so on, as appropriate).

Blood transfusions will be used to save life as an emergency measure, as a long-term attempt to arrest the deterioration of a vital organ and occasionally (but only as a temporary measure) to improve the quality of life, for example to reduce mother–baby separation resulting from frequent admissions to hospital, or to enhance wellbeing during a course of study or a much-needed holiday abroad. This treatment is embarked upon reluctantly, not only owing to the many commonly known risks of blood transfusion, but also because these people, as a result of repeated transfusions, may run into problems with iron overload and are particularly at risk of becoming untransfusable due to the accumulation of antibodies. This obviously has implications for pregnancy, as well as for long-term management and prognosis.

SERVICE PROVISION

For professionals to respond adequately to women with HbOs who are pregnant or seeking to become so, some essential services must be available. These include:

- laboratory services for diagnosis in adults and the fetus;
- genetic counselling services;
- expert medical care throughout life for the treatment of people with the disease states;
- psychotherapeutic counselling services to support individuals and their families, at any stage of life, with the many difficult emotions and adjustments with which they may have to deal.

Service providers need to be aware of the needs of clients and ensure that services meet these needs. Appropriate literature should be provided in the relevant languages. Counsellors must be acceptable to the clients. All staff must be rigorously educated about the dangers and implications of racism, for both themselves and their clients (Adams 1994).

SCREENING IN THE MATERNITY UNIT

Different maternity units have different policies depending on the population considered to be at risk and therefore needing to be screened. It is important to remember that all screening programmes have a percentage of failures (usually around 10–20 per cent) and that selective screening programmes are the most fallible. It is essential, therefore, for midwives to maintain an awareness of the relevance of screening for their clients throughout the entire reproductive process. They should not assume that, because screening tests were meant to have been carried out earlier, they have necessarily been done.

In an ideal world, everyone would know and understand their HbO status long before they embarked on a pregnancy, but this situation is still a long way off. At the booking visit, every woman who is likely to be at risk should be screened for HbO. Such an approach is however unlikely to be effective without extensive education of the relevant staff and 'at-risk' communities and careful administrative structures (Adjaye *et al.* 1989).

Some hospitals (such as St Thomas' in London) have developed units within the computerised booking package that request information about the country of origin of the woman, her parents and grandparents. Although this does not guarantee that every woman who is at risk of HbO will be identified, it has greatly increased this likelihood. Screening should also be offered to all partners who attend the booking appointment. This is only a beginning, however, as this information is quite worthless unless the appropriate response is made.

Normal results

Each woman who has been screened should be informed of her result and be given sufficient explanation to ensure that she can understand its significance and be reassured.

Unclear results

Difficulties in obtaining a definitive diagnosis for alpha and beta thalassaemia (which are often almost indistinguishable from iron deficiency anaemia) are not uncommon. It is, however, vital that a diagnosis is made in order to achieve an appropriate response. Genetic counselling must be provided for those with thalassaemias, and iron therapy for those with iron deficiency. Haematologists will advise on the additional blood tests needed to obtain clearer results. In the meantime, a sensitive balance must be maintained between dealing honestly with the woman and not making her unnecessarily anxious.

Positive results – women with traits

It is important that there are clear policies specifying the actions to be taken when a blood test result indicates a diagnosis of any trait. The aim of this response is to ensure that each woman obtains all the information, support and access to facilities that she needs and wishes. To ensure that this happens the following must be available.

Partner testing

The offer of screening for the woman's partner has the most likely benefit of demonstrating that he does not have an HbO and that the baby is therefore not at risk of inheriting a major HbO. The partner may, however, be unavailable or unwilling to be tested. If this is the case, it is important that encouragement to take the test is not at a cost of greater anxiety on the part of the woman, especially as women are, unfortunately, often not offered counselling unless both partners are known to have HbOs. If the partner's result is unknown, many women will need even more support than other women until the baby has been tested. Some partners may be encouraged to attend for testing if a simple letter explaining the request is provided. This should be given to the woman herself to avoid breaches of confidentiality, unless she specifically requests that it be sent directly to her partner.

Counselling

All women with an HbO should be offered an appointment for genetic counselling with a person trained in the specialty. If no trained HbO counsellor is available, referral should be arranged to a haematologist experienced in the management of HbOs, or to the nearest sickle cell and thalassaemia information centre, as a matter of urgency. In the meantime, information, support and realistic reassurance should be given.

Genetic counselling should include information about the nature and behaviour of the relevant HbO, the possible results of its interaction with other HbOs, a clear description of the choices open to the woman and referral for any requested procedures (such as chorionic villus sampling) or to other avenues of support. This must be done by trained counsellors who are able to provide this information free from personal bias. The object of this exercise is not that the woman does what the health professional thinks is best, but that she is enabled to make the best possible decision for herself, her baby and her family. Whatever the outcome, it is imperative that she experiences as much control over that choice as is possible.

SCREENING OF THE NEWBORN

There are two main reasons for screening for HbOs in the newborn. The first is to identify those babies with major HbOs and thus to be able to reduce the risks to them by providing the necessary medical care (see below). The second reason is to identify children with HbOs so that their parents can be informed and the family can be offered genetic counselling. It is essential to be able to ensure that adequate follow-up is available and provided, although this is not always the case (Milne 1990).

The risk of sudden and preventable death in infants with sickle cell disease is significant. Early diagnosis and institution of prophylactic measures can prevent this. It is imperative, therefore, that effective policies and procedures are in place to ensure the safety of these children (Eboh & van den Akker 1995). The authors' study at St Thomas' hospital demonstrated clearly the unreliability of selective screening. This unreliability appeared to increase as the selectivity increased. For example, screening all black women produced a 7 per cent failure rate but screening all babies of black women with traits produced a failure rate of 20–30 per cent. Selective screening also places great responsibility on the midwife. In spite of frequent claims to the contrary, usefully reliable results can be obtained from cord blood by a committed and experienced laboratory. Some units are now using the Guthrie spot for HbO testing. This has the benefit of using a tried and tested collection system, although even the Guthrie testing is likely to show a failure rate. All tests should be repeated (usually at 3 months), but the early test means that the baby's status is identified, the parents can be informed and therefore the baby's chances of receiving the appropriate follow-up are increased. The early diagnosis means also that there is a sufficiently long time to educate and counsel parents before there is any danger of the baby becoming ill. It is a tragedy to lose this opportunity.

Babies with traits

The baby's HbO status remains the same for life. It is sensible therefore to have a system for communicating this information to the health visitor and family doctor. This can be done via routine discharge papers, employing special standard format letters. All neonatal HbO results could be sent to the Child Health Records Department, which could be briefed to relay them to the appropriate health visitor. If such an arrangement is instituted, it is important that parents are informed of it.

Although few health authorities have the resources to provide counselling to every family, it is imperative that suitable literature is available, with contact addresses of organisations from which additional information can be obtained.

It is important that the baby's HbO status is known so that every attempt can be made to ensure as healthy a life as possible for the growing child. Medical problems encountered by children with sickle cell disease are discussed below. The families of babies with traits will need to be aware of the implications for any other children they may have, and indeed for the children that their child may have in the fullness of time.

Babies with a major HbO

Ideally, each parent of an affected child will not only be aware that a major HbO is a possibility before the baby is born, but will have already met the HbO counsellor. However, the real world is not always quite like this.

Parents should be informed as soon as possible after the diagnosis is made, by a person confident about the information who is able to provide appropriate counselling. Shock, denial, depression and anger are all normal responses. An intensive follow-up counselling programme must be available and must include the repetition of information already given, as well as a place for coming to terms with the difficult feelings involved. This must be sensitively provided in response to the needs of the family. Each member of the team must behave towards the parents with understanding. Parents of children with special needs frequently report the distress caused by the insensitive behaviour of others. They rarely wish for the subject to be ignored, or to be blindly 'reassured', or to be advised 'not to think about it'. It is nearly always possible to acknowledge that one is aware of the news, offering an opportunity to talk, and it is kind to do so. One does not have to be very knowledgeable, as just listening quietly and

with acceptance is valuable. People have different needs for companion-
ship and solitude at different times, and withdrawal does not always mean
that a person wishes to be left alone.

In spite of the enormity of the news for the parents, the baby is not at
any risk from its blood disorder at this stage. At birth, and for at least 4
months, babies are protected by their fetal Hb. It is not until they are about
4–6 months post-term, when they switch to making their adult version of
Hb (which in their case will be HbSS or some other combination) that they
are at risk. As far as their HbO is concerned, they can be treated exactly the
same as any other baby. Guilt, grief, anger and other feelings may make
this difficult for the parents to appreciate, but it can be helpful to have this
pointed out.

Children with sickle cell disease are likely to be at particular risk from
overwhelming septicaemia, most often caused by pneumococcal infection
to which their antibody response is greatly impaired, and from splenic
sequestration. Both of these events can cause death in a matter of hours.
However, they are entirely preventable through the simple measures of
penicillin prophylaxis throughout childhood and by teaching mothers the
signs to look out for. Mothers can be taught to palpate the spleen, the
consequent early warning resulting in a dramatic reduction in mortality
from this complication. These two measures illustrate the vital importance
and benefit of the early diagnosis of these conditions.

PREGNANCY AND SICKLE CELL DISEASE

Early papers on this subject suggested that patients not only had reduced
fertility, but were also more likely to spontaneously abort, have small
babies and show raised perinatal and maternal mortality rates (Serjeant
1985). Although more optimistic figures are now available, it is clear that
pregnancy is a hazard for these and their babies (Konotey-Ahulu
1991; Howard & Tuck 1995). It is also very unpredictable and the quality
of maternity care may be a crucial factor (Adams 1994). Pregnancy may
also have a deleterious effect on the woman's symptoms, and life-threatening events may be more common (Serjeant 1985; El-Shafei *et al.* 1992;
Howard & Tuck 1995).

There are also significant risks to the fetus. Miscarriage (in around 19
per cent of pregnancies), premature labour, low birthweight (in approxi-
mately 31 per cent of babies) and raised perinatal mortality have all been
reported (El-Shafei *et al.* 1992; Brown *et al.* 1994; Howard & Tuck 1995).
Brown *et al.* (1994) found the most common complications in fetuses and
newborns with sickle cell disease to be jaundice (25 per cent), fetal distress
(13 per cent), anaemia (10 per cent) and respiratory distress (6 per cent).
It is of paramount importance, therefore, that those caring for women
whose pregnancies are complicated by sickle cell disease are well informed,

meticulous in their observations and sensitive to their clients' individual concerns and needs.

These pregnancies must be supervised by an experienced team comprising midwives, haematologists, obstetricians and an HbO counsellor. The woman's haematological and obstetric progress must be carefully monitored throughout the pregnancy, particular attention being paid to any changes in her general health and the development of her baby. In addition to other obstetric care, Doppler velocimetry (ultrasound) may be helpful in early detection of babies at risk of low birthweight (Billett *et al.* 1993).

Medical factors can be particularly closely intertwined with social and psychological factors in this disease. Stress affects the circulatory system in ways that make sickling more likely to occur. This is commonly misunderstood, and patients are likely to be accused of coming into hospital 'just because they've got problems at home'. They may well have problems at home, but now they are in hospital as well. Help must be provided to resolve those problems if the woman's health is to improve. It is therefore imperative that a holistic approach is used and referral to and liaison with other agencies fully implemented. To fail to do this is to fail the woman and jeopardise her health and her baby's future. All aspects must be closely monitored in order to ensure the best possible outcome for the woman and her baby.

THE ROLE OF THE MIDWIFE

The midwife has a crucial role in the care of women with HbOs. In caring for those with a chronic illness, it is important to remember that they have a significant history with their illness within the health care system, and that they often know more about their illness and what they need than do many of their carers. Past experiences may have left them ambivalent towards health professionals, and repeated periods of hospitalisation may make them reluctant to attend clinics unless it cannot be avoided. In addition, having sickle cell disease may have had an important impact on a person's self-image, beliefs, self-efficacy, relationships and support structures (Leavel & Ford 1983; Morgan & Jackson 1986; Gil *et al.* 1989; Midence & Shand 1992). It is vital that a good, trusting relationship with the woman is initiated as early as possible, and that every effort is made to ensure the appropriateness of her care.

It must be remembered that the woman with sickle cell disease has limited energy that must not be wasted by inefficient systems; hospital appointments, for example, must be arranged to coincide whenever possible. She needs to understand why her lifetime pattern of care might now have to be changed. She must be enabled to feel confident about pathways of admission, and how to obtain advice about any concern she may have regarding herself or the baby.

Many people with sickle cell disease tend to postpone hospital admission until the last possible moment. A woman who is not pregnant and who is familiar with her own body will not usually be placing herself in serious danger by this approach. During pregnancy, however, the situation is different. Both the severity and the speed of onset of a crisis during pregnancy may catch the woman unawares, endangering her own life and/or that of her baby. She therefore needs to understand the requirement for earlier presentation, and efforts must be made to encourage her to do so.

Preconception care

Genetic counselling should ideally be provided long before reproduction is embarked upon, so that the woman is aware of her own and her partner's blood test result and the possibilities for their children. Where a pregnancy has been planned, it is much more likely to commence with the woman in possession of all necessary information of the possible courses and outcomes. Unfortunately, this is not always the case (Howard *et al.* 1993).

If there is a risk of the baby having a serious HbO, the mother should be counselled by a trained HbO counsellor to elicit her feelings and wishes regarding prenatal diagnosis and termination. There is no 'right' or 'wrong' decision. What is important is the opportunity for informed choice on the part of the parents. An additional consideration for a woman with sickle cell disorder who is considering prenatal diagnosis is the stress of looking after a sick child when her own health is not good, and the effect on her and the baby of repeated separations due to the illness of one or the other.

The booking visit

A careful history must be taken, as always, with special attention being paid to the family history of sickle cell disease and other illnesses. It is not at all uncommon for women to have lost other children with sickle cell disease, or to have sisters, cousins or friends who have died of it, sometimes during pregnancy or the puerperium. This is bound to have a profound effect on the woman's confidence, increasing her anxiety, and should be sensitively borne in mind throughout her care.

It can be most useful at this point also to obtain a history regarding the usual course of the woman's illness. This can provide a useful comparison later when trying to gauge the effect of the pregnancy on the course of her condition. A deteriorating picture will indicate the need for more intensive observations, or even intervention. This could be medical but may be simply a matter of support to make life less stressful. All concerns should be immediately and aggressively responded to, as there is rarely a place for 'wait and see'.

Partners should be tested at this stage, if this has not already been arranged, but it must be remembered that if the partner is unavailable, anxiety may be caused by the suggestion of testing. The most common benefit of knowing the partner's Hb status is that if he does not have an HbO, there is reassurance that the baby will not be seriously affected.

Sources of support

The booking visit is not too soon to discuss the support upon which the woman will be able to call after the baby is born. This needs to be re-examined throughout the pregnancy as her circumstances may change. At the booking visit, it is important to identify any possible shortfalls and begin at once to address these by working with her and other agencies. Caring for a new baby is an exhausting job for anyone, but it poses an additional strain on the precarious health of women with a sickle cell disorder. If catastrophes and potentially disastrous early separations of mother and baby are to be avoided, extra support may well be needed, and early planning for this provision is essential.

The woman's current social situation also needs to be explored. Poor or insecure housing can have a deleterious effect on her health, as can financial worries, poor diet and insufficient rest. Referral to a social worker should be made and the importance of these issues made clear. Strong letters to official bodies, such as housing departments, made by a health professional can be extremely effective, and midwives should consider writing them; persuading the consultant to countersign them may further increase their impact.

The need for additional blood tests should be discussed with the haematologists so as to avoid unnecessary venepuncture. Venous access is precious and venepuncture unpleasant.

Follow-up visits

The woman should be seen at each visit by a consultant obstetrician or a senior registrar experienced in the care of sickle cell pregnancies (Serjeant 1985; El-Shafei *et al.* 1992). Continuity is especially important with such women, as the signs of deteriorating health may be quite subtle and may be missed or ignored by someone unfamiliar with the condition or the patient.

Being more than usually susceptible to infection, women with sickle cell disease are especially prone to urinary tract infections (Serjeant 1985). These can make them extremely ill and must be diagnosed and treated as soon as possible. A midstream specimen of urine should therefore be obtained at each visit.

There is a low threshold for action if intrauterine growth retardation is suspected (El-Shafei *et al.* 1992; Brown *et al.* 1994; Howard & Tuck 1995), and regular Doppler scans should be carried out.

Blood transfusions

There is a seemingly endless debate regarding the relative value of blood transfusion in pregnancy (Koshy & Burd 1991; Howard 1994). Not only does blood transfusion carry the risk of introducing infection, but repeated transfusions may in addition cause accumulation of antibodies in the recipient, which will eventually render her untransfusable. Largely agreed criteria for recommending transfusion would seem to be deterioration in maternal health, life-threatening events, twins or a catastrophe in a previous pregnancy. Each case must be considered individually, although there are a few centres where blood transfusions are offered routinely to all pregnant women with sickle cell disease.

Crises

The most common crisis to occur is the painful bone crisis. This is rarely dangerous but is an indicator of ill health and, more importantly to the patients, can cause excruciating pain, for which enormous doses of analgesia are required. It is commonplace for doses of pethidine as high as 200 mg 2 hourly to be required for days or even weeks at a time, causing great anxiety to carers. The current literature does not identify drug dependency in the neonates of women with sickle cell disease. This may be due to the reduced risk of physical dependency when the drugs are used appropriately, that is, to control pain. Accusations and/or threats of 'addiction' are among the most common and distressing experiences for people with sickle cell disease and are often made by ill-informed people at times of immense personal distress for the person concerned.

Labour and delivery

Labour is a time of extreme vulnerability for a woman with sickle cell disease. Stress, both physical and psychological, hypoxia, dehydration and changes in body temperature are all likely occurrences in any labour and are the very situations most liable to precipitate a crisis. In addition to this, the woman may have deep and unexpressed fears about the risks to her own and her baby's life.

It is of paramount importance to form a trusting relationship with the woman as soon as possible and to take every opportunity to offer reassurance. Midwives are often reluctant to address the concrete fears of the women they care for, and find it hard to know how to do this, but it would be cruel to ignore these fears. It is easy to ask, 'Are you scared?' Whatever the answer, this can be followed up with a clear statement that although it is understandable to be frightened, the woman is not in danger, and that you, her midwife, are taking personal responsibility for her safety. Details of what measures are being taken to ensure she is safe should then be given.

Koshy and Burd (1991) have suggested that labour should be managed as for a patient with congestive heart failure. The following are vital considerations.

1. *Adequate analgesia.* This is important in order to reduce stress and maintain trust. It must be remembered that the woman may have a lifelong and tortured relationship with pain, and that she may have some level of tolerance to analgesics, thus requiring higher doses than would normally be expected. Epidural analgesia is effective and encouraged for these women.
2. *Oxygen therapy.* Many centres prescribe this routinely, but it is certain that there should be a low threshold for its initiation.
3. *Hydration.* Dehydration must be avoided at all costs. Again, many centres set up intravenous therapy regimes at the onset of labour. It may be possible to maintain adequate hydration by the oral route, but in view of the copious amounts required, the intravenous route is probably necessary. Renal damage, leading to an inability to concentrate the urine, means that an oral intake in excess of 3 l per day is required in normal circumstances. Drinks should be fresh and acceptable – 3–4 l per day of tepid tap water is not pleasant! It must be remembered that fluid intake and output should be closely monitored.
4. *Fetal monitoring.* Perinatal morbidity and mortality rates are significantly raised in these cases, so fetal monitoring should be continuous and meticulous.

As long as there are no contraindications, a vaginal delivery is preferable. Pelvic contracture, however, is a risk in these women, resulting in cephalopelvic disproportion. Should a caesarean section be necessary, postoperative care should be as for any other woman – early mobilisation, adequate analgesia and sufficient rest.

The puerperium

Postnatal care is the same as for other women, with the proviso that the midwife is aware of potential problems and is prepared to take any necessary action earlier rather than later. Many women with sickle cell disease are well during labour and the first few postnatal days, only to become seriously ill between the fourth and seventh days. This process is not fully understood but may be a delayed manifestation of the stress of the labour, the result of an untreated infection, a response to hormonal changes or the effect of the exhausting work of caring for a new baby.

For this reason, it is necessary to practise the utmost vigilance while caring for the woman and to provide as much help as possible with the baby. A single room may also enable the woman to obtain more rest. A woman with sickle cell disease should never be discharged home before the seventh day, and then only if both she and the baby are completely well. Home visits by an experienced community midwife who is aware of the issues should, at minimum, be made at least once a day until the 14th day.

Throughout this period, attention should be paid to the mother's general health and energy, any signs of infection or slow healing and whether she has any pain. Before discharge, the midwife should ensure that adequate support is available, and if it is not, social services should be informed and encouraged to help.

Contraception

Oral contraceptives are often withheld from women with sickle cell disease in the belief that the medication is dangerous for them (Howard *et al.* 1993). However, there is little or no evidence for this belief, and the real risks of a pregnancy for these women must be remembered. The theoretical risks of oral contraceptives do not constitute sufficient reason to withhold them from women for whom they are the most appropriate method of contraception (Serjeant 1985).

Intrauterine devices are also often discouraged because they are thought to cause infection. There is no evidence of an increased rate of intrauterine infection in women with sickle cell disease (Serjeant 1985), but it might be advisable to bear in mind that any infection might have rather more serious consequences for these women.

Many women are now using condoms, as they provide protection from sexually transmitted infections as well as pregnancy. They can, however, be unreliable, as can other barrier methods. Depot preparations of medroxyprogesterone acetate can be a useful and effective contraceptive, as its absorption is not affected by gastrointestinal disturbances, to which this group of patients is prone. It has also been suggested that it might have a beneficial effect on the course of sickle cell disease and thus might have the dual benefit of providing both effective contraception and an improvement in the woman's health (Serjeant 1985).

For permanent contraception, tubal ligation is the procedure of choice if a permanent male partner is unwilling to undergo vasectomy.

Contraception is an important issue for a woman with sickle cell disease, and any decision that she makes should be the result of correctly informed choice (Howard *et al.* 1993).

THALASSAEMIAS

There are two common forms of thalassaemia: alpha thalassaemia (A thal) and beta thalassaemia (B thal), affecting the production of alpha- and beta-globin chains respectively. Fewer chains are made, so less total Hb can be made. On routine blood tests, A thal traits have a picture almost identical to that of iron deficiency, with which they are commonly confused. It is vital, however, to differentiate between these two conditions if correct responses are to be made. People with A or B thal trait require expert genetic counselling.

Babies who inherit A thal from both parents are unable to make either adult or fetal Hb. This is incompatible with fetal life, and the baby is usually born prematurely as a hydrops fetalis or stillbirth.

If B thal is inherited from both parents (beta thalassaemia major), the baby will be unable to make any adult Hb. This is obviously incompatible with life, and the individual will need blood transfusions for life. In addition to this, iron chelation therapy will be required to prevent the life-threatening complications of the resulting iron overload. Currently, the only way of undertaking this is by subcutaneous transfusion, which takes about 12 hours a day, 6 days a week throughout life. It is therefore vital to obtain a correct diagnosis so that these families can be given the opportunity of receiving all the information and support that they require.

SUMMARY

Sickle cell disease and thalassaemia are inherited abnormalities of Hb manufacture. They affect every aspect of the sufferer's life. This is particularly pertinent during pregnancy when all women, not only those with additional health problems, have additional needs for understanding and support.

All women at risk of having inherited an HbO should be offered preconception and genetic counselling. If they are already pregnant, antenatal testing with appropriate counselling follow-up must be offered.

All pregnant women with sickle cell disease should be regarded as being at 'high risk' during pregnancy, as should their unborn children. The midwifery challenge is to provide responsive, woman-centred care to this special client group. The midwife must develop a trusting and empathic relationship with the woman as early as possible and monitor her complex and changing needs. She should take every opportunity to empower the woman and facilitate informed choice. She should acknowledge that the woman herself is likely to be an expert on her own medical condition and should respect her accordingly. In addition, she must have the courage to learn to address the issues pertinent to her patients, such as racism or the fear of dying or losing the baby, so that real trust can exist, and reassurance and comfort be given.

The midwife must be aware of the obstetric and medical complications to which the woman may be prone. She should bring all her skills of observation to bear and be vigilant for signs of problems. Once the woman is discharged back into the community, midwives and social service staff should be made fully aware of her situation.

Discharge from midwifery care is not an end – it is only the beginning of the mother's and baby's life together. If one or both are prone to serious illness, there will be many difficulties to be encountered. Midwives have the privilege of being in a position to facilitate a good relationship between them in the early days, in order to sustain them through the difficult times – this too is part of the midwifery challenge.

Acknowledgement

I would like to express my deep respect and gratitude to all the people affected by haemoglobinopathies with whom I have had the opportunity to work. I thank them for their patience, courage and humour in their dealings with me and with their situation, for teaching me all the really important things that I needed to know about haemoglobinopathies, for continuing to forgive my inadequacy and impotence, and for being a ceaseless inspiration to me in my life.

REFERENCES

Adams S 1994 Sickle cell disease: a case to answer? *British Journal of Midwifery* **2**(10): 475–8

Adjaye N, Bain BJ, Steer P 1989 Prediction and diagnosis of sickling disorders in neonates. *Archives of Disease in Childhood* **64**:39–43

Billet HH, Langer O, Regan OT, Merkatz I, Anyaegbunam A 1993 Doppler velocimetry in pregnant patients with sickle cell anaemia. *American Journal of Hematology* **42**:305–8

Brown AK, Sleeper LA, Pegelow CH *et al.* 1994 The influence of infant and maternal sickle cell disease on birth outcome and neonatal course. *Archives of Pediatrics and Adolescent Medicine* **148**(11):1156–62

Eboh W, van den Akker O 1995 Service provision for sickle cell disease. *British Journal of Midwifery* **3**(4):189–90

El-Shafei AM, Dhalawal JK, Sandhu AK 1992 Pregnancy and sickle cell disease in Bahrain. *British Journal of Obstetrics and Gynaecology* **99**:101–4

Gil KM, Abrams MR, Phillips G, Keefe FJ 1989 Sickle cell disease pain: relation of coping strategies to adjustment. *Journal of Consulting and Clinical Psychology* **57**(6):725–34

Horn MEC, Dick MC, Frost B *et al.* 1986 Neonatal screening for sickle cell diseases in Camberwell: results and recommendations of a two year study. *British Medical Journal* **292**:737–40

Howard RJ 1994 Blood transfusion in pregnancies complicated by maternal sickle cell disease. *Contemporary Reviews in Obstetrics and Gynaecology* **6**(3):117–21

Howard RJ, Tuck SM 1995 Sickle cell disease and pregnancy. *Current Obstetrics and Gynaecology* **5**(1):36–40

Howard RJ, Lillis C, Tuck SM 1993 Contraceptives, counselling and pregnancy in women with sickle cell disease. *British Medical Journal* **306**:1735–7

Konotey-Ahulu FID 1991 *The Sickle Cell Disease Patient.* London: Macmillan

Koshy M, Burd L 1991 Management of pregnancy in sickle cell syndromes. *Hematology/Oncology Clinics of North America* **5**(3):585–96

Leavel SR, Ford C 1983 Psychopathology in patients with sickle cell disease. *Psychosomatics* **24**(1):23–37

Midence K, Shand P 1992 Family and social issues in sickle cell disease. *Health Visitor* **65**(12): 441–3

Milne RIG 1990 Assessment of care of children with sickle cell disease: implications for neonatal screening programmes. *British Medical Journal* **300**:371–4

Morgan SA, Jackson J 1986 Psychological and social concomitants of sickle cell anaemia in adolescents. *Journal of Paediatric Psychology* **11**(3):429–40

Serjeant GR 1985 *Sickle Cell Disease.* Oxford: Oxford Medical Publications

FURTHER READING

Adams S 1994 Sickle cell disease: a case to answer? *British Journal of Midwifery* **2**(10): 475–8

Anionwu EN 1983 Screening and counselling in the antenatal and neonatal period, Parts 1 and 2. *Midwife, Health Visitor and Community Nurse* **19**:402–6, 440–3

Anionwu EN 1991 A mutli-ethnic approach. *Nursing* **4**(41):12–45

Brown M 1994 Mothers with sickle cell disease. *Health Professional Digest* **3**:5–6

Eboh W, van den Akker O 1995 Service provision for sickle cell disease. *British Journal of Midwifery* **3**(4):189–90

Modell B 1990 The ethics of prenatal diagnosis and genetic counselling. *World Health Forum* **11**:179–87

Williams J 1990 The Second Leicestershire Conference on Sickle Cell Anaemia and Thalassaemia. MIDIRS Information Pack no. 15, December 1990. Bristol: MIDIRS

Midwifery care for travellers

Mandy Churcher

In recent years, sensational reporting by the media and the government response to travellers have raised the profile of this heterogeneous group of people. The aims of this chapter are, first, to consider travelling women within their social context and, second, to explore how midwives might offer appropriate care as indicated by an examination of health care issues and research evidence.

During the antenatal, intrapartum and postnatal periods, a travelling woman has the same needs as any other woman. It is anticipated that an understanding of the particular context of the travellers' culture and lifestyle will help the midwife to offer appropriate care.

For the purposes of this chapter, the term 'travellers' will include all travelling people, gypsies and tinkers, and, generally, a distinction between 'new' travellers and other travellers will not be drawn. A definition by Hussey (1990) enables one development of a broader perspective: 'people who may or may not share a language... but who do have a commitment to a life that is similar'.

There are a number of projects across the country seeking to meet the challenges of providing health care to travellers (Eckford 1990; Rose 1993; Tyler 1993; J. Wilkins, personal communication, 1993). However, although there is a growing body of literature by health care professionals, there is a dearth of midwifery-specific sources. Yet the midwife, too, is part of the multidisciplinary team who will be involved in offering care to women and their families.

TRAVELLERS WITHIN THEIR SOCIAL CONTEXT

Effective discussion of midwifery care provision for travellers is impossible without first exploring the context of care.

A problem of definition

Liegeois (1987) suggests the framework of four distinct traveller groups in the UK:

- North Welsh Kale
- South Western and English Romanichals
- Irish Parees and Minciers
- Scottish travellers.

The 1968 Caravan Sites Act includes 'Persons of nomadic habit of life whatever their face or origin' but it does not include 'members of an organised group of travelling showmen, or persons engaged in travelling together as such'. This definition is restated in the Criminal Justice and Public Order Act (1994) and obviously excludes certain people who would identify themselves as 'travellers'.

There is a notion that somehow there is a true-blooded gypsy and that others have merely appropriated the term. The romantic image applied to the Romanies may result in a stereotype that dehumanises them and labels them as exotic. This may cause them to be viewed as separate and alien from the wider population but also lends strength to the concept of the true and traditional traveller – in contrast to others who 'sponge' and 'scrounge' off society (Bates 1989). This has been highlighted particularly by the 'new' travellers who are not seen as 'real' or genuine travellers. Hawes and Perez (1995, p 8) suggest that it is not possible to 'discuss Gypsy issues without acknowledging that large numbers of people who live in caravans do not conform to the generally accepted notions of what is meant by that term'.

Although it is true that there are some culturally specific areas for some groups, many of the issues that face any traveller are similar. More than a third of local authorities would evict a newly delivered woman from an unauthorised site (Fletcher 1993), and in some areas women are not immune from harassment even when they are in labour (Sadler 1993).

In response to findings from the Maternity Alliance concerning the health of travelling women, a group of individuals from Save the Children Fund and other interested parties set up the 'Safe Childbirth for Travellers' campaign in 1990. The primary focus was to stop the eviction of pregnant and newly delivered women from sites and to ensure that local authorities were aware of the health circumstances of travelling families and took the needs of pregnant women, mothers and babies into account before considering eviction. This forward-thinking campaign anticipated the Criminal Justice and Public Order Act, which received Royal Assent on 3 November 1994. The 1968 Caravan Sites Act, whereby local authorities had a duty to provide sites for travellers, was repealed.

Local authorities may now use their discretion with regard to site provision and maintenance. Central government funding for site provision and maintenance is no longer available, and local authority and police powers to stop unauthorised camping as well as the number of eviction orders, without recourse to the court, have increased (Lloyd 1994; Maternity

Action 1995; MIDIRS 1995). With a reduction in site provision, it is felt that homelessness and imprisonment for failure to comply with eviction orders may increase (Davis *et al.* 1994). Access to health care may further be reduced and the statutory duties of the Children Act (1989) may not be fulfilled. The UN Committee on the Convention of Children's Rights in 1995 considered that the Act would have a major impact on the rights of gypsies and travellers.

However, guidelines from the Department of the Environment, entitled 'Gypsy Sites Policy and Unauthorised Camping' (DoE 1994) may be used in dealing with local authorities when travelling clients in their care are faced with possible eviction. Point 9 of these guidelines suggests that local authorities 'should use their powers in a humane and compassionate fashion'. Point 13 states, 'When deciding to proceed with an eviction, they should liaise with relevant statutory agencies, particularly where pregnant women or newly born children are involved, to ensure that those agencies are not prevented from fulfilling their obligations towards these persons'.

In September 1995, eviction procedures were challenged by a group of travellers in Lincolnshire and Sussex. Mr Justice Stalley ruled that Wealden District Council and Lincolnshire County Council were 'legally wrong in failing to take account of the human factor' (Gibb 1995). Proper enquiry into the needs of travelling people, including pregnant women, was not made before evicting them, and the eviction order was overturned in the Wealden case.

Safe Childbirth for Travellers is persistently refocusing the campaign but would wish to monitor the effects of the 1995 Act on the case of women and their children. A positive strategy is for midwives to give appropriate information to the campaign; their address can be found at the end of the chapter. They can also be contacted for help and information.

Reduced access to maternity care is not purely a geographical concept but may be due to ineffective communication. There is evidence that travellers are considered to be a deviant group and are on the receiving end of active discrimination (Kenrick & Puxon 1972; Okely 1983; Feder 1989; Durward 1990). An awareness of travelling people and their individual perspectives is vital for any midwife providing care. More information about their culture might decrease discrimination and improve the standard of health care provided (Feder 1989).

History

Okely (1983) tells us that 'The history of the Gypsies is marked by attempts to exercise, disperse, control, assimilate or destroy them'. In Europe, there was a general belief that they brought death and disease (Kenrick & Puxon 1972). Although there was a theory that they originated in Egypt, records of travellers in England have been known since the sixteenth century.

Henry VIII ordered their expulsion, and those who did not leave were judged as felons and executed.

In the Second World War, they were branded as 'antisocials' and more than 250 000 were executed by the Nazis. More recently, they have been the victims of 'ethnic cleansing' in Romania (Bridge 1993).

In England, Wales and Scotland, there are thought to be around 12 000 'caravans' or household groups, but this may be an underestimation (Fletcher 1993). The most common geographical areas of habitation are East Anglia, Kent, Wales, Scotland, London and urban areas of the Midlands.

Cultural issues

For some established travelling people, there are common factors that may affect their lifestyle, health and acceptability of health care.

Travelling people generally have a different attitude to work from that found in the wider society. Preferring to be self-employed, they see work as something to be integrated into their lifestyle – although the recession has brought constraints to their working patterns. Helping with seasonal farm work and calling on houses has been replaced by scrap metal dealing, manual work on the roads, carpet selling and even landscape gardening (Okely 1983; E. Fletcher, personal communication, 1993). However, there is an increase in the numbers of men on income support and of women being 'trailer bound'. Since travelling people live alongside, yet independently of, the wider society, this loss of their own employment has been disempowering. This has led to an increase in alcoholism, smoking and marital disharmony (Crout 1987). Investment of resources is in items that may easily be exchanged for cash (such as jewellery or cars) and definitely not in building societies or banks.

The travelling society is close knit, and strong ties are made through kinship and marriage. It is, in essence, also a patriarchal society. The outsider, called the 'giorgio', is viewed with suspicion, and it may be salutary to realise that the giorgio may be considered as dirty or polluting (Okely 1983).

It is generally expected that women will marry early and be pregnant within 18 months (Raper 1986). In the past, families were large, but this is changing. Research in Avon 1990–2 found that the main reasons for reduced family size were physical exhaustion and financial hardship (Hawes & Perez 1995).

Living conditions

The trailer is nearly always scrupulously clean, even though the quality and size will vary. Better trailers may have coal fires, while others may have poor insulation and Calor gas heating, leading to condensation. Travellers choose to live in a trailer and may have a mobile lifestyle. Taking up residence in a house is normally due to shortage of sites, rather than through choice.

Where there is a problem with sites, some travelling families may be housed in bed and breakfast hostels or other buildings. It seems that public housing options are not easily obtained (Davis *et al.* 1994). Living in a house may impose difficulties and restrictions not encountered in a caravan, and adjusting to the differences may be hard. Some travellers appear to find the space overwhelming, choosing to live in one room only. Repairs may provoke anxieties – it is not possible to take a broken window from a house to be mended as it is with a trailer window.

Hygiene rules are described by Okely (1983). These reflect the way in which travellers live and their view of the giorgio, and go some considerable way to explaining why they see house-dwellers as dirty. The outside is seen as a covering for the inside, and anything internal must be clean. This is expressed in the belief that polluting dirt may be visible yet must be separate. Therefore the site need not necessarily be tidy and clean, but the inside of the caravan must. There is a definite system for ensuring that washing of the body, clothes and cooking utensils are undertaken in separate places in the caravan, as well as in separate bowls. Kate, a travelling woman, describes the system:

> We have a clean bowl to wash up in, a different bowl to wash our face in and a different bowl to wash our clothes in. Inside toilets are thought to be polluting and therefore often not used in the trailer. In the past, menstruating women and those who have given birth were also considered to be polluting.

According to Fletcher (1993), if a death occurs the trailer must be burnt and the family must move on. On a settled site, this may mean moving pitches.

Travellers and the giorgio

There is an uneasy relationship between travellers and the wider society. Hostility is frequently directed towards travellers, their presence in an area is seen to 'lower the tone' and there are many examples of open aggression towards them (Save the Children Fund 1992). Constant eviction from sites and threats and fears of abuse are not uncommon.

Given the pervasive and deeply rooted mistrust, it is hardly surprising that travellers do not readily accept outsiders and that their policy should be that 'it is safest to mistrust giorgios'. For midwifery care to succeed, there needs to be outreach on the part of the midwife, enabling a movement from distrust through knowledge to a degree of mutual understanding. Midwives need to begin by attempting to understand why the distrust is there in the first place.

The 1993 Midwives' Rules state that 'The continued attendance of a midwife on a mother and baby is requisite' for a minimum of 10 days and a maximum of 28. Post delivery, women must be visited on site. The challenge implicit in visiting travelling women is to optimise their care provision, and a midwife who has already built up a relationship with a woman is likely to be able to provide better care than one who has not. Although not always easy to achieve, this aim can be facilitated through continuity of care.

Site provision

Provision of sites may vary in quality and there is a shortfall. The impact of the Criminal Justice Bill has yet to be fully revealed, but site provision is a key issue for the travellers' lifestyle and health. Permanent sites, which have bathroom and washing facilities per pitch, may not be without drawbacks. Travellers who might not normally choose to live together find themselves on the same site – which may lead to tensions and difficulties. Even official sites, such as the one described below, have been shown to be inadequate in various amenities:

> Regulations state that there should be only one caravan per pitch, but every pitch has two, sometimes three, caravans. There are large banks of rubble and soil dividing up the site and the caravans. Children use them as play areas while family pets and other animals use the banks as places to deposit excreta. (Batstone 1993)

HEALTH ISSUES

Many sources quote poor general health issues. Environmental aspects are detrimental to health (Riverside HA 1992). Smoking may be common (Riverside HA 1992), and alcoholism and obesity may be problematic (Crout 1987). The sites themselves may be environmentally unfriendly and less than ideal for women who have tiny babies or who are pregnant. Amenities may be limited, and the lack of basic requirements such as water or toilet facilities compound the difficulties for both the women themselves and the professionals caring for them.

The Northern Gypsy Survey (1993) interviewed 63 families and found that 45 per cent requested improved sanitation and 37 per cent felt that moving regularly affected their health care.

Lack of knowledge about general health issues and bodily awareness in women is common. Their poor understanding of their bodies may lead to misunderstandings of health issues. However, it is generally felt that one-to-one work, through designated health workers, is gradually changing the situation.

Travellers themselves state their needs as being secure, safe sites with sanitation, water supplies and freedom from environmental problems. Health needs are secondary to these more pressing ones (Feder 1990). This raises the issue of the focus of 'health care' research, which may fail to look at the real issues and lead to victim blaming and further stereotyping.

Maternal and child health

In 1988, Pahl and Vaile published their results of interviews undertaken by health visitors in Kent on 263 mothers, all with at least one child under the age of 15 years. The women had had 814 pregnancies in all. The results demonstrated a dissatisfaction with site provision, 14 per cent having no mains water supply, 21 per cent no mains elecricity and 33 per cent no toilets. Only 6 per cent of the women stated that they had not been ill in the previous 5 years. Among the sample, 55 per cent had received no antenatal care when pregnant, 97 per cent had delivered in hospital and the majority of deliveries were normal. Low birthweight occurred in 12.8 per cent of the sample. The stillbirth and neonatal death rates (per 1000 total births) were 12.0 and 16.0 respectively. These figures are above the national average, but the study has been criticised since there was no way to verify the self-reporting (Feder 1989). Furthermore, health visitors working with travellers report no unusual incidence of low birthweight or raised complications in childhood (L. Dodge, personal communication, 1993; E. Fletcher, personal communication, 1993).

The Association of Metropolitan Authorities (AMA) surveyed its 67 member authorities on their policy towards the eviction of pregnant women in July–October 1988. Of 43 respondents, 16 said they would evict pregnant women, 13 would evict women close to birth, and 15 would evict mothers with a newborn baby (Durward 1990).

Among the cases collected by Save the Children Fund is that of Mary, 19 years old, $7^1/2$ months pregnant and living on an unauthorised site. The local council decided to evict the travellers, although the land was derelict. The travellers decided to move on before being evicted, and eventually Mary moved up north to be near friends. For the last part of her journey, she was in labour and, for the delivery, had to go to an unfamiliar hospital (Morton 1992). Another case from the same collection is that of a young woman in late pregnancy and unwell, waiting for an ambulance to take her to hospital, who was meanwhile barricaded in by the local council with earth mounds that caused severe problems with access (Morton 1992).

Moving on in pregnancy is not only stressful but also means that the woman may not be able to visit the hospital where she has been booked or achieve any form of continuity of care (Sadler 1993). This may reinforce the commonly held view of travellers as being deviant, non-compliant and uncaring about their unborn child. They are seen either as 'late bookers' or as poor attenders, 'defaulters'. Compounding this situation is the difficulty of not having a postal address at which they might be contacted. Furthermore, it should not be assumed that all travelling women can necessarily read.

The midwife should know what action she can take as the woman's advocate to prevent eviction or to ensure that services are provided. She can contact the local authority and ask for a pregnant or recently delivered woman not to be evicted or moved on, by using the Department of Environment guidelines (DoE 1994) (Fletcher 1993). She can also contact the environmental health officer to ensure that services will be provided as legally required (MIDIRS 1995). An example of a midwife acting on her client's behalf is given by Harold (1993). The client was on Forestry Commission land and wished to have a home delivery. The Forestry Commission wished to evict the woman, but the midwife acted as her advocate and negotiated with the Commission's personnel, thereby forestalling the eviction until after the woman had delivered.

Access to care has been highlighted as problematic for many women (Department of Health 1993). Furthermore, the Chief Medical Officer has stated that the NHS must take positive steps to eliminate discrimination (Calman 1992). Some positive steps to address this challenge might include:

- redirection of resources from high-tech hospitals to community care – more midwives who are able to provide care in the community and facilitate travelling women to use existing services;
- legislation to protect pregnant women and newly delivered mothers from eviction;
- a friendly reception in hospital and clinics and a real attempt 'to understand and not to try and change their ways' (S. Salter, personal communication, 1993)
- provision of health promotion information in an acceptable format.

Access includes not only knowing where to go and being physically present but also involves the interaction that takes place between the caregiver and the client. It is all too possible for a spiral of poor communication to occur. Take, for example, the woman who, despite having been born in England, had a strong Southern Irish accent. She had previously delivered a baby at the hospital where she was booking for the second time. The receptionist at the antenatal clinic told that woman that she would not be entitled to NHS treatment. Despite her protests about having been born in England, she was sent a bill for £1895 following the birth of the baby. Her communication skills had been insufficient to argue her case and the receptionist had acted in a judgemental way. One of the challenges facing midwives is that of establishing how such situations can be prevented.

MIDWIFERY ISSUES

The woman's position is clearly defined by many travellers, and there are certain issues which are a woman's domain. If a midwife seeks to discuss 'taboo' issues with the men, she should expect to encounter hostility and possibly rejection. It is quite normal for the men to disappear from the caravan when the midwife comes to visit – this should not be taken as a sign of unfriendliness. Many travelling women view pregnancy as their private business, not to be discussed by other members of the community (L. Dodge, personal communication, 1993; E. Fletcher, personal communication, 1993). For this reason, visiting women on site may be perceived as eroding confidentiality, and many women may find a locally based 'drop in' service preferable.

Continuity of care

If continuity of care is to be an achievable aim, the midwife's role in liaising with other health professionals becomes the more important when clients are moving site on a regular basis. Many authorities have health visitors and social workers who are designated to work with travelling people. Since they cross boundaries that midwives do not, their relationship with the travellers may be more firmly established. Some GPs are also known among travelling people to be sympathetic to their cause (Feder 1990). If this is the case, midwives should not miss opportunities for liaising with them.

It is generally recognised that it takes time to build a relationship with travelling people. The development of trust is unlikely to be facilitated by constant change (E. Fletcher, personal communication, 1993). As midwives tend to work for one health authority, they will have problems maintaining continuity when travellers move around. Where sites are more permanent, however, allocating responsibility for travelling women and their babies to one midwife or a small team of midwives has proved to be successful (L. Dodge, A. Eckford, J. Wilkins, personal communications, 1993).

Communication by health care workers may be facilitated by hand-held notes. Family record cards with information about the GP, social services, vaccinations and immunisations, cervical smear status and any disabilities in the family have been introduced by Batstone (1993) to improve communication. The use of hand-held notes (Feder 1990) has been a positive development in empowering travelling people.

Certain investigations, for example cervical smear tests, may be refused by some clients. Some travelling women find the use of a vaginal speculum unacceptable. Termination of pregnancy is often seen as an unacceptable option among travelling peoples, so blood tests designed for detecting abnormality may be refused.

Care during pregnancy

Antenatal care may not be valued: booking into a hospital is for the purpose of securing a bed for delivery (Milne 1988). Education by health visitors has improved the uptake of antenatal care and, where this is provided in a friendly setting in which travelling women are accepted, it would appear that uptake is appropriate (J. Wilkins, personal communication, 1993).

If a woman does not keep an antenatal appointment, it is vital that she is not viewed as deviant or 'a defaulter'. She may be travelling. The letter may not have reached her, especially if her site is not a permanent one. She may have received the letter but be unable to read it. If a woman must be contacted, and the appearance of a uniformed midwife might breach confidentiality or cause alarm, it is advisable to contact the health visitor and ask her to make the visit.

Similarly, travelling women may not attend parent education classes. However, this can be carried out to a degree on an individual basis during antenatal appointments.

The birth

Childbirth was traditionally seen as polluting and took place at the edge of the camp (Okely 1983). This view is still held to varying degrees, and most births now appear to take place in hospital. Men do not generally stay with their women during labour (Raper 1986). Some women are extremely frightened by the hospital environment (J. Wilkins, personal communication, 1993); the strangeness and fear that hospitals may engender in this group of women mean that it is particularly important that midwives employ all their skills to help make the experience of childbirth a positive one. Knowledge and understanding will enable the removal of stereotypical images that some midwives may use to make judgements about the different care that women want. These judgements themselves are a factor in the inequality of health provision (Bowler 1993).

For some 'new' travellers, birth in the home situation is considered to be the ideal, and there are instances of midwives undertaking home deliveries in caravans and teepees (Blake & Langford 1988; Dodson 1990). A study undertaken in Avon found that of 82 women, 38 delivered in maternity units in Avon, 3 had home confinements and for the rest no record of their delivery existed owing to travelling (Hawes & Perez 1995).

Generally, the community will respond to the baby's arrival by visiting the hospital in large numbers. Many women, however, wish to return home as soon as possible. Midwives may have difficulty actually finding their clients if the address given when the woman leaves hospital is that of a temporary site.

Care in the postnatal period

The demands on the woman to look after other children are likely to be high, and it may not be easy for her to rest. The midwife's role in supporting her is as important as for any other postnatal woman, but support is particularly pertinent with some specific areas of maternal and infant health.

Maternal infections, including breast abscesses and vaginal infections, are not uncommon. Stress incontinence and dyspareunia are cited by health visitors as common difficulties. The support, advice and information a midwife gives may reduce this morbidity. This may be through listening to the client, offering advice or referring the woman to other agencies.

The issue of contraception is important. This should never be discussed if others are present – it is more appropriate to ask, 'May I have a word with you?' Different methods of contraception are acceptable to different individuals. Generally, barrier methods are not acceptable to either sex, and natural family planning is rarely practised. The oral contraceptive pill and Depo-Provera are becoming more acceptable to many women, as is the intrauterine contraceptive device. The choice will depend upon the client's motivation towards different methods, although the younger women are certainly likely to discuss contraception in the right setting (Morton 1988).

It is likely that many travelling women have chronic levels of depression (Crout 1987), which may be due in part to the constantly insecure environment in which they live. A midwife who has developed a good rapport with a woman may be able to counsel and support her.

Where infants are bottle fed, a significant role for the midwife is to ensure that the mother is able to reconstitute and store the feeds correctly. Gastrointestinal and oral candida infections are common, demonstrating the need for education about sterilisation of feeding equipment. Heating in poorly insulated caravans may be by Calor gas which causes problems with condensation, and may lead to chest infections. Fear of hypothermia causes some women to overwrap their baby, thereby increasing the risk of sudden infant death. Health education on this issue is vital therefore.

There is a reported higher incidence of genetic conditions among travelling families, often due to intermarriage (Batstone 1993). In 1991, Gordon *et al.* surveyed 203 families in Ireland and found 12 cases of congenital abnormality among 350 children. The abnormalities detected were congenital talipes (3 cases), coarctation of the aorta (1), congenital glaucoma (2), renal abnormalities (2), coeliac disease (2), I-cell disease (1) and Hurler's syndrome (1). There was a high level of consanguinity among this population, a risk factor also detected by Tyfield *et al.* (1989), who studied phenylketonuria in a Welsh travelling family. However, some groups are now discouraging the marriage of first cousins, which is a positive strategy to prevent such a high level of abnormality occurring (A. Eckford, personal communication, 1993). Travellers will always care for their children – adoption and child abuse appear to be rare.

SUMMARY

During the continuum of childbirth, travelling women will benefit from the support of a midwife they have come to know and trust. Recent changes in the maternity services, and the emphases on continuity of care and accessibility of services, should enable more travelling women to receive this benefit.

Midwives should ensure that they know the specialist professionals (health visitors, local authority officers and social workers) designated to work with travellers in their own area. They should be aware of which GPs in the area are sympathetic towards travellers.

Midwives should be aware of whom to contact if there is an environmental problem with a site they are visiting, and should be familiar with the appropriate strategies to employ if an eviction order is being placed on a site where a pregnant or newly delivered woman is living. Individual MPs, the local authority and the Safe Childbirth for Travellers campaign can all be contacted about issues concerning site provision.

In areas where travellers are seen regularly, midwives could evaluate the way in which midwifery care is provided to travelling women. How is continuity of care achieved? Would it be appropriate to change working patterns so that a small team of midwives is responsible for visiting the women?

A real challenge for midwives is to make themselves as aware as possible of the women's multicultural perspective, to be respectful and non-judgemental, and to seek to provide an appropriate service that will maximise the chances of any individual travelling woman receiving the best possible care. An informed and individual approach may lead to improved access to health care and outcomes for travelling women and their babies. It may lead to midwives acting as catalysts for change at local (and possibly at government) level as they seek to bring about change by active representation of travelling people.

REFERENCES

Bates D 1989 Travellers and Education in Inner London. Unpublished dissertation held at the Institute of Education, London

Batstone J 1993 Meeting the health needs of Gypsies. *Nursing Standard* **7**(7):30–2

Blake J, Langford J 1988 Midwife to the hippies. *Midwives Chronicle* **10**(1211): 382–3

Bowler I 1993 They're not the same as us: midwives' stereotypes of South Asian descent maternity patients. *Sociology of Health and Illness* **15**(2): 157–77

Bridge A 1993 Romanians vent hatred against Gypsies. *The Independent* 19/10/93, p 13

Calman KC 1992 *On the state of the public health 1991.* The Annual Report of the Chief Medical Officer of the Department of Health for the year 1991. London: HMSO

Crout E 1987 Trailer bound. *Community Outlook* May:12–14

Davis J, Grant R, Locke A 1994 *Out of site, out of mind.* London: Children's Society

Department of the Environment 1994 *Gypsy Sites Policy and Unauthorised Camping.* DoE circular 18/94. London: HMSO

Department of Health 1993 *Changing Childbirth, A Report of the Expert Maternity Group.* London: HMSO

Dodson L 1990 Happy alternatives. *Nursing Times* **86** (10):40–2

Durward L (ed.) 1990 *Traveller Mothers and Babies: Who cares for their health?* London: Maternity Alliance

Eckford A 1990 On the road. *Health Visitor* **3**:204–5

Feder G 1989 Traveller Gypsies and primary care. *Journal of the Royal College of General Practitioners* **39** (327):425–9

Feder G 1990 The politics of traveller health research. *Critical Public Health* **3**:10–13

Fletcher E 1993 Safe childbirth for travellers. *Professional care of Mother and Child* **3**(1):6

Gibb G 1995 New Age Travellers win ruling against eviction. *The Times* 1/9/95, p 2

Gordon M, Gorman DR, Hashem S, Stewart DGT 1991 The health of travellers' children in northern England. *Public Health* **105**:387–91

Harold J 1993 Correspondence. *Maternity Action* 60 (May/June): 4

Hawes D, Perez B 1995 *The Gypsy and the State.* Bristol: Salis

Hussey R 1990 Regional Health Seminar Report, to be found at the King's Fund Library, London

Kenrick D, Puxon G 1972 *The Destiny of Europe's Gypsies.* Sussex University Press, in association with Heinemann Education Books, London

Liegeois JP 1987 School Provision for Gypsy and Traveller Children – orientation document for reflection and action. European Economic Community, Paris. Distributed by Traveller Education Service, Manchester

Lloyd L 1994 The Criminal Justice Bill: Implications for midwifery practice. *British Journal of Midwifery* **2**(11):559–61

Maternity Action 1995 Travellers' hopes dashed. *Maternity Action* **65**:11

MIDIRS 1995 Travelling families. *MIDIRS Midwifery Digest* **5**(4):481–2

Milne C 1988 Mobilising health care. *Nursing Standard* **2**(34):22–3

Morton J 1988 Control of fertility amongst travellers. *Midwife Health Visitor and Community Nurse* **24**(8):314–16

Morton J 1992 Case histories held by Save The Children Fund, London

Northern Gypsy Survey 1993 From Myth to Reality. Copies can be obtained from the Northern Gypsy Survey

Okely J 1983 *The Traveller Gypsies*. Cambridge: Cambridge University Press

Pahl I, Vaile M 1988 Health and health care among travellers. *Journal of Social Policy* **17**(2):195–213

Raper M 1986 Travelling families in Northumberland. *Health Visitor* **59**:345–7

Riverside HA 1992 *Travellers Health. Riverside District Case Study No. 14.* London: Public Health Directorate, Riverside HA

Rose V 1993 On the road. *Nursing Times* **89**(33):26–7

Sadler C 1993 Out in the cold. *Nursing Times* **89**(16):16–17

Tyfield LA, Merideth AL, Osbourn MJ, Harper PS 1989 Identification of the haplotype pattern associated with the mutant PFU allele in the Gypsy population of Wales. *Journal of Medical Genetics* **26**(8):499–503

Tyler C 1993 Traveller's tale. *Nursing Times* **89**(33):27–31

FURTHER READING

Adams B, Okely J, Morgan D 1975 *Gypsies and Government Policy in England.* London: Heinemann

Beckingham A 1992 Who falls through the net? *Community Care* **11**(3):13–14

Billington T 1986 GP to the hippie convoy. *General Practitioner* 8/8/86, p 11

Chambers J 1991 The impact of a music festival on local health services. *Health Trends* **23**(2):122–3

Reid T 1993 Partners in care. *Nursing Times* **89**(33):28–9

Richardson PJ 1989 Travelling folk. *Journal of the Royal Society of Health* **109**(5):181–2

USEFUL ADDRESS

Safe Childbirth for Travellers
6 Westgate Street
Hackney
London E8 3RN   Tel: 0181–533 2002

The hidden abnormality: the birth of a child with a previously undiagnosed handicap

Karen Connolly

This chapter was inspired by the personal experience of the birth of a child with an undiagnosed congenital abnormality and by professional experience of supporting women coming to terms with this situation.

The chapter describes what might be considered 'normal psychological responses' to birth, in order to understand more fully the ways in which women and their partners may respond when faced with the birth of a child who does not fulfil their expectations. If the midwife is aware of the possible responses, she is more likely to be able to help, as well as being more likely to help herself to cope with a particularly stressful part of her role.

A POSITIVE VISION OF PARENTHOOD

Pregnancy and childbirth are listed as 'major life events' (Holmes & Rahe 1967) and as peak developmental experiences by psychologists (Rappoport *et al.* 1977). The outcome will therefore have far-reaching effects on all concerned. The birth should be essentially joyous, but it may be marred for several reasons, not least because the baby is abnormal.

Today, in the Western world, women are usually able to choose when to have a baby. Many women have the opportunity to benefit from contraceptive advice, fertility treatment, antenatal screening and, should the fetus not be perfect, the opportunity to terminate the pregnancy. Thus expectations are likely to be very high. Women imagine that they will give birth safely to a live and healthy baby, at the appropriate time.

For a small percentage of women, this dream is shattered when they give birth to a baby who is less than perfect. How parents accept and learn to cope with this new situation can be greatly affected by the professionals, especially midwives, obstetricians and paediatricians.

BEFORE CONCEPTION

The motivation for having a baby has been well documented (Raphael-Leff 1991) and may include attaining adulthood, building a family, passing on one's genes and having someone to love, as well as a response to social and cultural pressures. Or the pregnancy may be unplanned. Once conception has taken place, however, the woman will experience a variety of physical changes and undergo a series of social and emotional adaptations in anticipation of childbirth. Some women will view this as a period of development, others as a time of crisis (Romney 1984). No matter how much the child is wanted, the woman has to become accustomed to the idea of this 'being' sharing her inner space and part of her inner world (Raphael-Leff 1991). Many women will feel that the pregnancy takes over their life and find that they are planning the future for both themselves and the baby.

The family relationships will alter, together with wider social networks, as the woman and her partner anticipate the responsibilities of parenthood. These may be, at the same time, both demanding and joyful, daunting and satisfying (Ball 1987).

Preoccupation with the pregnancy may explain the vivid dreams experienced by many women and why one aspect of such dreams is often the baby's normality. We would do well to remember that different cultures have different definitions of what is 'normal'. The Siriono of Bolivia, for example, nurture babies with congenital talipes equinovarus but regard twins as unnatural (Mead & Newton 1967). The availability of modern screening methods, of termination for fetal abnormality and of techniques to treat the fetus even before birth may well have affected the view of what is 'normal' in our own culture.

MOTHERHOOD MEANS CHANGE

The impending birth of the first child constitutes the greatest life change that most women will ever have experienced (Kitzinger 1994). They have to consider the effect that motherhood will have on their careers and other aspects of their lifestyle. Changes in body shape can profoundly affect a woman's sense of self-worth, especially with regard to how attractive she feels her partner finds her.

Couples who considered their communication to be good prior to conception may find a deterioration following the birth. There may be emotional outbursts, periods of inattention for each other and an inability to support each other as before (Romney 1984; Kitzinger 1994). Relationships must change as individuals move into another phase of their lives. Furthermore, the changing nature of families today means that few women have the support of a larger extended family. Frequently, social support to ease the transition to parenthood is lacking (Raphael-Leff 1991).

Media pictures of motherhood and new babies tend to be glamorised, the negative aspects being ignored or minimised. Foster (1995) brings to our attention an advertisement from a private fertility clinic, which glamorises motherhood as follows:

> There is no other perfume like it, the smell of the newborn: a milk scent, warm scent cuddle essence.

As a result, many mothers feel guilty if they find their new baby difficult to bond with (even though the process of 'attachment' is rarely instant or straightforward – for a fuller discussion, see Salariya 1990). They can feel even worse if the changes to their lifestyle seem at first overwhelming. And yet expectations may have been so unrealistic. In the Western world, where most births take place in hospital, many women will only have seen 'newborn' babies as depicted by the media. The babies of friends, seen at home after a little time and several baths (and without the weight of responsibility), will be very different from a newly delivered baby, still unwashed and unwrapped.

FATHERHOOD

The role of the father varies from culture to culture, but fatherhood is a social construction as the man has none of his partner's physical changes to identify him as a parent-to-be (Summersgill 1993). During the pregnancy, however, he will find his own way in which to adapt. A percentage of fathers may even display symptoms of pregnancy (Fawcett 1978; Summersgill 1993). On the other hand, the father's response may be less positive. He will see his partner change, both physically and psychologically, and he is still expected to attend favourably to her needs. He is expected to react supportively and sympathetically when she has mood swings and when she becomes excessively tired and finds difficulty in moving. The father's role requires new skills, but there is little support available to him. Is it any great wonder then that some men find that the increased demands, perhaps in the face of a reduced income, together with other stresses, such as (in some cases) a reduced libido on the part of his partner, all combine to make the prospect of parenting rather more trouble than it is worth?

SIBLINGS

The reaction of older children to a new baby may vary depending on previous preparation, parental attitudes and experiences, as well as the child's age and temperament.

What the child begrudges the unwanted intruder and rival is not only the suckling but all the other signs of maternal care. It feels that it has been dethroned, despoiled, prejudiced in its rights; it casts a jealous hatred upon the new baby and develops a grievance against the faithless mother. (Freud 1933, cited in Raphael-Leff 1991)

The sibling's reaction may be further complicated if the baby is born with a congenital abnormality. The older child has to cope with the burden this places on the parents, both physically and emotionally. He or she is often in danger of becoming the 'forgotten' member of the family, whose need for support goes unheeded (Trause & Irving 1983, cited in Raphael-Leff 1991). Kennedy (1985) noted that the siblings of handicapped children can be bitter over the attention lavished on the disabled child and the accompanying social discomfort, including stares from strangers and teasing or taunting from friends. These children may, therefore, require help and counselling in order to help them cope with their family situation.

UNDETECTED ABNORMALITY

Despite the fact that there are many antenatal investigations available to detect fetal abnormality, still some babies are born with a previously undetected abnormality.

Estimates of the total incidence of congenital abnormalities vary widely depending upon what is regarded as serious enough to include and up to what age the infants surveyed are followed. Many defects may not become apparent until middle or late childhood. On average, however, a congenital abnormality of significance occurs about once in every 30 live and still births; in 25% of these babies there is more than one defect. Minor abnormalities occur in about another 3% of total births. (Johnston 1994, p 153)

GRIEF AND ADJUSTMENT

The period immediately following the birth is crucial. This is often when the parents first learn of their baby's abnormality, and when, by whom and how they are told are all extremely important. Common questions asked at the time of birth are, 'Is it a boy or a girl?', 'How much does it weigh?' and 'Is it all right?' It is the response to this last question that begins the process of realisation and adjustment for the parents.

As discussed earlier, parental hopes and expectations are likely to have been high during the period leading up to the birth. Together, they may have imagined what their child would be like and hoped that it would be healthy, beautiful, bright and loving. There may have been hopes that the child would resolve family discord, enforce wedlock, be the one to carry on the family name and even be better in every way than the parents. The birth of an imperfect baby takes away all these idealistic hopes, leaving the parents both disappointed and devastated. They will need to grieve for the baby they did not have, as well as come to terms with the one they did have.

The parents will be subject to a vast range of emotions, including bewilderment, disbelief, guilt, shame and humiliation. These are all part of a pattern of adjustment described by Klaus and Kennell (1983), which is effectively a process of mourning and resolution as described by a number of authors (Kubler-Ross 1970; Drotar *et al.* 1975; Romney 1984). Most writers agree that the first stage is one of overwhelming shock in which the sufferer feels helpless and tearful. This can last days, weeks or even months. It is followed by a period of disbelief and denial. The parents have an urge to flee from the situation or awaken from a bad dream. A further stage is one of sadness, anger and anxiety, in which the parents may have long periods of crying and feeling angry with themselves or with the infant, hoping that the baby will die. Some mothers, believing that death is imminent, actively reject the baby in the hope that this will protect them from further pain. The stages do not follow in any logical order. Parents can move on to anger, then back to disbelief, and then on again to attachment and rejection. The pain is inevitable and real.

Over the following few weeks and months, many parents will find a level of equilibrium as the intensity of their emotional reactions and anxiety lessens. Confidence in their ability to care for their child will gradually increase. The fifth and final stage of reaction to the birth of their child is one of reorganisation and adjustment, when the parents attempt to deal with the responsibilities of having a child with a congenital abnormality. They may by now have a more positive long-term acceptance. Mutual support increases in many cases, although, for some, the stress and strain is too much and leads to separation (Drotar *et al.* 1975).

According to Mercer's (1977) description of this grieving process, the parents may also experience a weakened self-identity and feel social stigma in having an abnormal child. The loss of the perfect child they never had, with the associated emotional and financial burdens, may be overwhelming. Parents will often attempt to gain as much information as possible about the defect in order to be able to deal with its reality. Socially, they may redefine themselves in their new role as the parents of a child with an abnormality. These social and cognitive responses described by Mercer are crucial in order to maintain and increase their self-esteem and to continue in society adjusted to their new role as parents.

ATTACHMENT

The terms 'bonding' and 'attachment' have been used over the past two decades to describe the process by which infant and mother become mutually interactive and aware. The adjustments contributing to this process have been overstated and frequently misinterpreted (Sluckin *et al.* 1983; Salariya 1990).

Kennell *et al.*, who in 1974 put forward the contentious claim that the first 3 days of life can influence the maternal–infant relationship over the course of a full year, later identified certain aspects of congenital abnormality that may affect the attachment of parents to their infants. These are as follows:

- Is the malformation completely correctable or is it non-correctable?
- Is it visible or non-visible?
- Is it life-threatening?
- Will it have an effect on the future development of the child?
- Is it a single or multiple malformation?
- Is it familial?
- Are there other members of the family with a defect?
- Does it affect the central nervous system?
- Does it affect the genitalia?
- Will there be a need for hospitalisation?
- Will repeated visits to the doctor or other agencies be required?

The importance of these aspects in relation to the bonding process was also noted by Romney (1984). However, when Sluckin *et al.*(1983) reviewed maternal attachment to infants with physical or mental abnormalities, they could find no conclusive evidence that there was any difference compared with the attachment to infants with no handicap. They found both mothers who were resentful and rejecting, and mothers who were loving and devoted. Perhaps it would be more helpful to be less concerned with measurement of levels of attachment very early on and be more aware of how far along the adjustment process between shock and acceptance the parent is at the time that the level of attachment is assessed.

THE ROLE OF THE MIDWIFE

The role of the professional may be crucial in determining the outcome in terms of speed of adjustment and subsequent emotional health. Professional caregivers, therefore, need to develop insight into and understanding of the psychological needs of their clients, and will ideally receive the same insight and understanding of their own psychological needs, as caregivers in stressful circumstances, from their colleagues.

Each midwife is personally accountable for her practice and should 'work in a collaborative and co-operative manner with health care professionals and others involved in providing care, and recognise and respect their particular contributions within the care team' (UKCC 1992). 'Each woman being cared for by a midwife should therefore obtain optimum care, since the midwife is working as a member of a multidisciplinary team where there is mutual understanding, trust, respect and co-operation' (UKCC 1989).

Coping and growing

When a mother is expecting a baby with a known abnormality, the professionals who are involved in her care can be both informed and prepared for the baby's arrival, and to some extent at least will have been able to forewarn the parents. The midwife looking after the mother will be experienced and, ideally, will have already established a relationship with this mother during the pregnancy. However, when a baby with an unexpected abnormality is born, neither the midwife nor the parents are prepared. The shock and disbelief of the parents may also be felt by the midwife. The reactions of the midwife will be watched closely and, according to McCarthy (1984), are remembered clearly by the mother for years after.

Some forms of congenital abnormality, such as a cleft lip, may be obvious to the parents at the time of delivery, in which case they are likely to want immediate information. Other abnormalities may be obvious only to the midwife, so she may have time to examine the baby carefully before approaching the parents. When the midwife has recognised that there is an abnormality, the manner in which this news is conveyed to the parents is very important. Those parents who see their baby's abnormality themselves should be given honest and reliable information to the best of the midwife's knowledge and be reassured that she will ask the paediatrician to come and see the baby and parents to give them more information. The midwife must admit that she does not know about all conditions and so must only tell the parents what she does know and reassure them that she will find out more. This is the beginning of a trusting relationship that will help the parents to trust other health care professionals. Parental disappointment may be displayed in many ways and can be distressing for the midwife involved. She should know that their reaction is normal and encourage them to express their feelings as they go through the various stages of adjustment. This is very important if they are to grow to love and accept their baby (Klaus & Kennell 1982). The role of the midwife, in standing alongside the parents as they express their anger, fear, distress and disappointment, is extremely important. She can help the parents to begin to accept their child. By supporting them, understanding their emotions and being non-judgemental, she can have a positive influence on parental attachment and self-confidence.

Communication

Parents should be told about the abnormality in appropriate terms, and medical jargon should be avoided. The midwife should be present when the doctor discusses the baby's condition in order to clarify any terminology used and to reaffirm what has been said. McMichael (1971) found that most parents wished to be told about their baby's condition as soon as it became apparent. The information must be accurate and up to date, and will need to be repeated and confirmed several times.

Communication is always difficult in times of stress. Shocked parents may resist unpalatable information. Sometimes information is quite consciously 'forgotten' because to remember it is too stressful. Hospitals, special care baby units (SCBUs) and other hostile environments become associated with fear and distress; in such environments, misinformation and confusion abounds.

Using a midwifery model, such as the assessment of needs model (Crichton 1992; Bryar 1995), helps the midwife systematically to address the woman's physical, psychological, spiritual and sociocultural needs. A clear record should be kept of what information and advice has been offered and what care has been given to this woman and baby. Conflicting advice is especially distressing and dangerous in this situation.

Support

The midwife should encourage the parents to see the baby as soon as possible, especially if the baby is ill and requires admission to SCBU or to the neonatal surgical unit (NNSU). Without this, they are liable to have a distorted image of the baby and its condition. If possible, the baby should be examined in front of the parents to highlight its normal features while allowing them to see the problems in relation to the baby as a full person. In this way, the midwife can behave towards the baby as she would any other and demonstrate to the parents that this baby is a person and an individual. The midwife, however, should not try to force attachment in parents who are not ready, as this may only serve to increase the doubt and guilt they may feel.

Midwives are well placed to counsel the parents, to allow them to talk and express their feelings. The midwife will have regular contact with the parents and will often be the one from whom they are most likely to seek advice. Klaus and Kennell (1982) stated that parents should be encouraged to talk in order to avoid becoming overwhelmed. This will enable them to gauge the reality of the situation. The midwife may therefore be the appropriate professional to co-ordinate the multidisciplinary team involved in the care of the baby. Regular meetings should be held involving all members of the team, including the parents, so that everyone is kept up to date. Parents should be given regular information so that they do not have to ask for it (Lynch 1989). Many aspects of care will involve decision making by the medical staff, but this should involve the parents. Penticuff (1988) stated that parents involved with severely ill babies should have a role in the treatment decisions as they are to live with the consequences for the rest of their lives.

Ethical dilemmas

Parents are considered competent to make these decisions when they are thinking rationally and fully understand their baby's condition and prognosis. However, the midwife should not make rash judgements on the parents' competency when they are emotional and employing defence mechanisms to cope with the crisis. They are still mourning the loss of their ideal child but, even so, may be able to make intelligent and rational decisions regarding their infant's care (Healy *et al.* 1985). By involving the parents in all aspects of such care, the midwife can help them to become confident and learn to accept the baby. It increases their self-esteem and proves they care for and love their baby (Solnit & Stark 1961). Ideally, this should be done at a pace dictated by the parents and not rushed or forced.

Ludman (1989), carried out a study that showed an increased incidence of depression and anxiety among mothers of sick term infants. This was due to a variety of factors, mainly because the mother was unable to carry out her normal caring role, and because of pressure from medical/midwifery staff for her to remain with her child at all times and resulting in further guilt if she did leave her baby, with its consequences for bonding.

Difficult decisions

Some parents may react to the birth of a handicapped child by saying that they cannot care for this baby and that they want it to be taken into residential care. This should be heard, understood and treated seriously. For some parents, such feelings form part of an initial reaction only; when they have learnt more about their baby and have been able to assimilate the information given to them, they will change their minds. However, some parents continue to feel that this is the only option open to them. Caring for this child appears to be more than they can cope with, for whatever reason. They may also have to deal with other factors, such as marital disharmony, sibling rivalry, altered career prospects and financial constraints. Such parents should be helped to talk through their decision and offered compassionate understanding while they try to decide what is best for both them and their child. These are major decisions with long-term consequences, and parents often need time to think carefully through the issues involved. At this stage, the child may be fostered, thus allowing the parents time to consider their decision.

MOVING ON

At some point, the parents will have to face other people – siblings, grand-parents or other relatives and friends. Some parents may feel isolated and reluctant to venture outside or let anyone see the baby. They may feel inad-equate, angry and guilty on the one hand, but on the other love the baby because of its helplessness (Solnit & Stark 1961). Midwives can help the parents to face up to this and can explain ways in which they can try to break the news to others. It may help to take the baby out and to be open in explaining the condition to their friends and relatives. This is often very difficult, and the first time can be the most emotional and even embar-rassing, but the more people are used to seeing them with the baby, the more acceptable it will be. As the mother and father have benefited by early contact with their baby, so will everyone else.

The parents may agree that involving others in the care of the baby will be helpful. The extended family and friends may provide welcome addi-tional support for the parents. The benefits of sharing are many, but if the mother or father becomes overprotective, the baby will miss opportunities to develop in a more balanced way and may become overdependent and subsequently more insecure. Again, the midwife can highlight ways in which the parents can stimulate the baby and allow normal behaviour patterns to develop. While the midwife's involvement with the parents is only for a relatively short period of time, she is present at a crucial time in the life of the family, one which may have profound effects on the way its members function together in the future, as well as on how they view other health care professionals.

Practical support

Support for this family with a handicapped child will need to continue for many years, so the family should be put in touch with the appropriate authorities as soon after the birth as possible. The midwife can act as co-ordinator between the various professions and other disciplines, and should have a good knowledge of each person's role. The 'Changing Child-birth' Report (Department of Health 1993) has laid down recommenda-tions for professionals when caring for parents whose baby is handicapped.

Before the midwife discharges the care of this family into the commu-nity (after 28 days, or longer if the baby is on SCBU or NNSU), she should ensure that the GP, social worker, health visitor and community nursing services are notified. Finances may become a burden to the family if the mother is not able to return to work, or the care of the baby may involve additional expenses over and above those usually incurred. Here, the midwife can arrange for the parents to see a social worker who will help the family claim any benefits to which they are entitled, and tell them of any charities (such as the Joseph Rowntree Trust) that may help with additional equipment needed for the home. In some areas, there is also a paediatric occupational therapy service, which will assess the needs of the child at home and any adaptations that may be necessary in the future. The midwife is legally responsible up to the 28th day after the birth, but during that time she can actually help the parents in many ways and can be a guide, friend and counsellor.

The parents need to be aware of the sources of support and help, especially in the early days when they are still suffering from shock. The NHS provides medical staff, nurses, midwives, health visitors, social workers, occupational therapists, psychotherapists, physiotherapists, play therapists and many others. There is also help and support from many other sources, including friends, families, lay support groups, self-help groups and the religious community. While the evidence in the literature (Glendinning 1983) suggests that most parents find such contact helpful, the midwife must be sensitive to the needs of parents who find such groups unhelpful and even disturbing. The midwife can help parents best by providing sources of information and contact names and addresses, and even by offering to accompany new parents to such groups. This help from a respected and trusted professional can have positive benefits for the parents and the child, both immediately and in the long term.

Professional support

There is much in the literature about loss and grief and how midwives as professionals can help women and their families to adjust to new situations (Mander 1994; Sherr 1995). To date, however, there is very little about the needs of the professionals who are deeply involved in caring for families at such a difficult time. Midwives will need help and support from their professional colleagues, either in the form of co-counselling or by established informal supportive networks. Time must be made available to care for the carers. Whatever mechanisms are employed to ensure that this help is made available, the need for its existence is beyond question.

Currently, most midwifery services are being run to try to ensure that women benefit from continuity of care, as highlighted in the report by the Maternity Services Select Committee (1992, the Winterton Report). Midwifery teams have been set up in some hospitals and communities, and where possible midwives aim to follow the women through the antenatal, intrapartum and postnatal periods. Such schemes allow midwives to develop closer relationships with the women and their families, but this sometimes does not allow the midwife any space to deal with her own emotions. Traditional methods of organising care, especially those that involve the allocation of tasks rather than people, provide ample opportunities for midwives to avoid too close an emotional contact. Where there is continuity of carer, support for the midwife assumes greater importance. When a midwife has been involved in the care of a woman and her family in which the outcome was poor, she needs to know that what she is feeling is normal. She may well experience feelings of shock, grief, self-doubt, anger and fear of the future. She may need to review what has happened over and over again in her mind. If the midwife receives good support, she will, after a period of time, put the emotion to one side and begin to reflect upon how she would deal with a similar situation again. She should then be able to accept the experience as one of learning, using it to teach others, retain her self-esteem and make personal progress. Making a record of the episode, how she dealt with it and what she has learned from it would be a valuable addition to the professional portfolio that all midwives are now advised to compile (UKCC 1991). When dealt with positively, such critical incidents are an important part of learning and growing professionally.

Peer support

What support is available to the midwife herself? The first port of call is probably her colleagues. Ideally, she should be able to discuss with them the events that have distressed her and how she feels about them. Thus her management of the case can be reviewed in a non-judgemental way, and she can be reassured that her feelings are normal and should be expressed.

Experienced staff should show those who are less experienced that the display of emotions is acceptable for professionals. Student nurses and midwives are taught about the grieving process in parents, and similarly it should also be acknowledged that professionals themselves sometimes need to grieve. The midwife should be encouraged to talk, as remaining silent will not help her to come to terms with her feelings. Caring for grieving parents can be very demanding, and the midwife directly involved will, where necessary, benefit from some assistance from her colleagues.

Ideally, a trained counsellor within each organisation should be available for both parents and staff alike. However, such a resource is often unavailable, and midwives, together with other health care professionals, try to counsel parents within the limits of their training and often with no emotional back-up. Midwives could actually help each other by listening and understanding, and should be prepared to suggest that a colleague sees a trained counsellor, via the GP, if that midwife is unable to come to terms with her emotional upset. She must not feel stigmatised.

Each midwife has a named supervisor of midwives to whom she can turn for support when faced with a situation that she has either not faced previously or in which she feels she needs help – be it personal or professional. The supervisor's role is not only to monitor the standards of midwifery practice, but also to be the midwife's guide and counsellor.

The practising midwife has responsibility for her own professional development. This was recognised by, for example, the English National Board on instituting the Framework and Higher Award in April 1992. This involved ten key characteristics that could be used by the midwife to identify her strengths and weaknesses. These not only help a midwife faced with a distressing situation, but would also assist the more experienced midwife to facilitate and assess the development of others (ENB 1990). Continuing education is a vital role in professional development.

SUMMARY

The psychological effects upon the mother, father and family following the birth of a handicapped baby are far reaching and longlasting. The arrival of the baby will affect all aspects of their lives for the foreseeable future.

Delivery of a child with a previously undiagnosed abnormality presents the midwife with a twofold challenge. First, she must support the parents in such a way that they are helped to come to terms with the reality of their situation. Second, and crucial for the first challenge to be met fully, she must accept that her own reactions of shock and devastation are natural, human emotions. The midwife must deal adequately with these, bringing into play all the professional skills at her disposal in order to achieve an equilibrium. Meeting these two challenges will enrich her own professional development, enhancing her ability to offer assistance to the family in their distress and helping them to accept and deal with their new situation.

The following should be remembered:

1. Ensure that you include topics such as counselling skills and coping with loss in the education you undertake in fulfilment of your statutory periodic refreshment requirement.
2. Listen to parents as they explore their initial grief. Do not attempt to give false reassurance, but give clear information when it is requested.
3. Make appropriate use of your supervisor of midwives, and learn to ask your colleagues for support when you need it.

REFERENCES

Ball JA 1987 *Reactions to Motherhood: The role of postnatal Care.* Cambridge: Cambridge University Press

Bryar R 1995 *Theory for Midwifery Practice.* Basingstoke: Macmillan

Crichton MA 1992 Assessment of Needs – Model for Midwifery Care. Unpublished dissertation for the MA Degree, Manchester University

Department of Health 1993 *Changing Childbirth. A Report of the Expert Maternity Group.* London: HMSO

Drotar D, Baskiewicz A, Irwin N *et al.* 1975 The adaptation of parents to the birth of an infant with a congenital malformation: a hypothetical model. *Paediatrics* **56**:711–17

English National Board for Nursing, Midwifery and Health Visiting (ENB) 1990 *Framework for Continuing Professional Education and Training for Nurses, Midwives and Health Visitors. Project Paper No. 3.* London: ENB

Fawcett J 1978 Body image and the pregnant couple. *Maternal–Child Nursing* **3**:227–33

Foster P 1995 *Women and the Health Care Industry: An Unhealthy Relationship?* Milton Keynes: Open University Press

Glendinning C 1983 *Unshared Care. Parents and their disabled children.* London: Routledge & Kegan Paul

Healy A, Keesee PD, Smith BS *et al.* 1985 *Early Services of Children with Special Needs: Transactions for family support.* Iowa: University of Iowa

Holmes TH, Rahe RH 1967 Social Readjustment Rating Scale. *Journal of Psychosomatic Research* **11**:219

Johnston PGB 1994 *Vulliamy's The Newborn Child.* Edinburgh: Churchill Livingstone

Kennedy H 1985 Growing up with a handicapped sibling. *Psychoanalytic Study of the Child* **40**:255–74

Kennell JH, Jerauld R *et al.* 1974 Maternal behaviour one year after early and extended post partum contact. *Developmental Medicine and Child Neurology* **16**:172–9

Kitzinger S 1994 *The Year after Childbirth.* Oxford: Oxford University Press

Klaus M, Kennell JH 1982 *Maternal–Infant Bonding.* St Louis: CV Mosby

Klaus M, Kennell JH 1983 Parent to infant bonding: setting the record straight. *Journal of Paediatrics* **10**:575–6

Kubler-Ross E 1970 *On Death and Dying.* New York: Macmillan

Ludman L 1989 The psychological care of mothers with very sick neonates. *Maternal and Child Health* **14**(7):197–9

Lynch ME 1989 Congenital defects: parental issues and nursing supports. *Journal of Perinatal Nursing* **2**(4):53–59

McCarthy T 1984 *The Physically Handicapped Child.* London: Faber & Faber

McMichael JK 1971 *Handicap: A study of physically handicapped children and their families.* London: Staples

Mander R 1994 *Loss and Bereavement in Childbearing.* Oxford: Blackwell Scientific

Maternity Services Select Committee 1992 *Health Committee Second Report, vol. 1, Report together with Appendices and the Proceedings of the Committee (the Winterton Report).* London: HMSO

Mead M, Newton N 1967 Childbearing: its social and psychological perspectives. As in Raphael-Leff J 1991 *Psychological Processes of Childbearing.* London: Chapman & Hall

Mercer RT 1977 *Nursing Care for Parents at Risk.* Thorofare, NJ: Charles B. Slack

Penticuff JH 1988 Neonatal intensive care: parental prerogatives. *Journal of Neonatal Nursing* **1**(3):77–86

Raphael-Leff J 1991 *Psychological Processes of Childbearing.* London: Chapman & Hall

Rappoport R, Rappoport N, Strelitz Z 1977 *Fathers, Mothers and Others.* London: Routledge & Kegan Paul

Romney MC 1984 Congenital defects: implications on family development and parenting. *Issues in Comprehensive Paediatric Nursing,* **7**(1):1–15

Salariya E 1990 Parental–infant attachment. In Alexander J, Levy V, Roch S (eds) *Postnatal care.* Basingstoke: Macmillan

Sherr L 1995 *The Psychology of Pregnancy and Childbearing.* Oxford: Blackwell Scientific

Sluckin W, Herbert M, Sluckin A 1983 *Maternal Bonding.* Oxford: Basil Blackwell

Solnit AJ, Stark MH 1961 Mourning and the birth of a defective child. *Psychoanalytical Study of the Child* **16**:523–37

Summersgill P 1993 Couvade – the retaliation of marginalised fathers. In Alexander J, Levy V, Roch S (eds) *Midwifery Practice: A research-based approach.* Basingstoke: Macmillan

Trause MA, Irving NA, 1983 Care of the sibling. In Raphael-Leff J (1991) *Psychological Processes of Childbearing.* London: Chapman & Hall

United Kingdom Central Council for Nurses, Midwives and Health Visitors (UKCC) 1989 *Exercising Accountability: A framework to assist nurses, midwives and health visitors to consider ethical aspects of professional practice.* London: UKCC

United Kingdom Central Council for Nurses, Midwives and Health Visitors (UKCC) 1991 *PREPP and You.* London: UKCC.

United Kingdom Central Council for Nurses, Midwives and Health Visitors (UKCC) 1992 *Code of Professional Conduct.* London: UKCC

FURTHER READING

McHaffie H 1994 *Holding On.* Hale: Books for Midwives Press
Stanton M 1992 *Cerebral Palsy: A practical guide.* London: Optima

USEFUL ADDRESSES

Contact a Family
170 Tottenham Court Road
London W1P 0HA   Tel: 0171-383 3555
                        Fax: 0171-383 0259

This organisation has a directory of over 900 support groups and can put families in touch with each other.

The Family Fund
Administered by the Joseph Rowntree Memorial Trust
PO Box 50
York YO1 2ZX   Tel: 01904 621115

CHAPTER FOUR

Them and us: poverty, deprivation and maternity care

Jean Davies

This chapter is based on work carried out in an inner city area in the north of England where long-term unemployment rates were high. Through working with some low-income women and their families, it became clear that the cultural impact of deprivation creates a divide between those on wages and those on welfare, between tax-paying professional and recipient – between them and us. This had an impact on how public services, including midwifery, were used. The work was an attempt to address some of these issues in the provision of a service that was effective, by being provided in a way that made it accessible.

There are many levels of economic division – Britain's poor would be considered rich by some living in other parts of the world; nevertheless, they are poor by the standards of the country in which they live, and the disparity between the upper and lower income ranges is increasing (Child Poverty Action Group 1996). Fortunately, unlike in other parts of the world (ICM 1993), mothers are unlikely to die as a result of childbirth, but the children in the lowest economic ranges have perinatal mortality and morbidity rates that are consistently higher than average (DHSS 1980a).

The effect of poverty on childbearing is one of the greatest challenges for midwifery care. While this chapter looks primarily at Britain, the international challenge of the effect of poverty needs to be kept in mind. Of the half a million women who die as a result of pregnancy and childbirth every year, 99 per cent of these deaths occur in developing countries (Downe 1991).

The title of this chapter is used as a way of emphasising that poverty divides not just in economic terms, but also in how social life is experienced. The Department of the Environment funded the Community Midwifery Care Project through inner city funding in Newcastle between 1983 and 1987 in recognition of the fact that special effort was needed to promote a better uptake of maternity care among low-income women (DHSS 1980a). Four midwives worked on the project, the aims of which were to evaluate the effectiveness of giving enhanced midwifery care to women considered to be at risk because of their socioeconomic circumstances. The evaluation was done by a social scientist, who was funded for the duration of the project.

The work continued in a modified way following the report of the project (Evans 1987); the evaluation showed that it was possible to give appropriate care to women whose economic circumstances place them in a category of risk. This, however, requires a recognition of what the needs actually are. Many of these were illustrated through the evaluation and research that was carried out as a follow-up.

The data for the Community Midwifery Care Project were gathered prospectively from 263 women who booked for maternity care in the course of 1 year. There were two control groups: a concurrent prospective study of women matched from hospital case notes, and a retrospective control of all the women from the study area who had delivered during the year before the project started. Data were collected through semistructured questionnaires, both pre- and postnatal, and also through case note review. Interviews were also taken with the professionals involved.

The four project midwives worked in a team in two areas of the city that were considered to have low-income indicators (DHSS 1980b). They had an average caseload of 60 women each per year. They gave enhanced care, which was defined as a minimum of four home visits, instead of the usual one. At these visits, diet and smoking were discussed, as were feeding and childcare. It was found that information given on a one-to-one basis was well received, and during these home visits many other issues came to light, often resulting in referrals to other agents such as social services departments. The midwives visited the women in hospital if they were admitted antenatally and also when they were in labour. Most of the deliveries were conducted by the labour ward staff, although the project midwives did deliver some women. Postnatal visiting was regular until the 10th day and extended to the 28th day. There was therefore continuity of carer throughout from a named and known midwife who was easy to contact in the community.

The most important aspect of the care was that it was community based and the midwives were easily accessible as in both areas they had local bases. The women attended their GPs and the hospital for antenatal care as usual, and the project midwives were aligned with GPs who worked in the areas. Some families had GPs from farther afield, and for these women the midwives provided a local point of contact. Local parentcraft classes were instigated in both the areas and the number of women who attended these was a reflection of the neighbourhood approach to the work, which not only made them accessible, but, by being focused locally, also made them more acceptable (DHSS 1986) (Table 4.1).

The importance of the work being locally based cannot be emphasised too greatly. As the midwives became familiar figures in the neighbourhood and through the local base, the number of informal exchanges increased and street 'consultations' were frequent. Early referrals for pregnancy became common as trust developed, and it was not uncommon for someone to stop a midwife on behalf of a neighbour or friend. The classes will be explored more fully below, as it was through these that it was possible to identify some of the particular issues relating to providing care in areas of economic deprivation.

Table 4.1   *Attendance at community-based parentcraft classes (reproduced from Evans 1987)*

Age	Project women (%)	Control women (%)
<20	38	9.3
20–30	24.6	5.5
>30	22.2	0
Attendance at hospital classes all ages		
All	4	9.8

The results of the work showed not only that women were very satisfied with the enhanced care they received, but that there were also positive clinical trends. Project women who had a previous preterm baby were shown to be less likely to have a subsequent preterm baby than the control women who had received no additional care.

Three-quarters of the project women smoked, but there was evidence that there was a greater reduction of smoking among project women during pregnancy than among control women. There was evidence from the postnatal questionnaires that the project women who received the additional information about nutrition had a greater awareness of nutrition, had improved their diet and maintained the modifications well into the postnatal period. The uptake of family planning and subsequent attendance at child health clinics was shown to be higher among the project women than the controls. Job satisfaction for the midwives was also raised.

THE PARENTCRAFT CLASSES

In one of the areas, the classes were run along traditional lines in the local clinic. The following relates to the other, which was run in a neighbourhood centre. This centre was a joint enterprise, set up by the project midwives and the social services department in order to provide health promotion through an attempt to increase self-awareness, confidence and esteem. The housing department provided a council house on the estate as the city council recognised that there were multivariate problems which it was hoped would be reduced through positive preventative measures.

The classes were hard to establish, as the women did not at first attend. Some of the men did not like it when they did and would come and say the women were needed at home; one man used to come outside the centre and whistle for his wife. Initially, the women were reminded in the morning that there was a class in the afternoon. These were presented more as a get together of those who were pregnant rather than as a class *per se*. It is not uncommon to experience difficulties in setting up classes in areas of high unemployment and low income, and the time involved in establishing them has to be considered if they are to succeed. Once they had been established, they developed their own momentum, as the women still wanted to come after they had had their babies. Out of this grew a children's centre, as the women not only identified the need for a meeting place, but, through the neighbourhood centre, were able to put together a case to the social services department for this to be developed.

The neighbourhood centre provided a non-clinical venue; eventually a steady flow of women attended and the group became known as 'Pregnant in Cowgate'. The aim was to give information about pregnancy, labour and parenting, and also about general health and childcare. The classes were unlike any experienced previously by the midwife who had had many years' experience in teaching antenatal classes. There was one vociferous woman who 'knew it all': she had four children, was having a fifth and would quite cheerfully tell the midwife, who only had three, that she was not as competent to talk about childbearing.

There was blunt realism, sometimes verging on the crude, as tales of events and happenings in the neighbourhood were told. These were considered more immediate than were discussions about babies, and out would pour dire tales the like of which this midwife had never heard; away the group would go on the wild whim of some local story, retold and elaborated, which centred on some activity that was quite often on the other side of the law.

Discussion about issues relating to pregnancy did take place but not in the way in which antenatal classes are usually conducted. It is a challenge to midwives to provide parentcraft education for client groups for whom structured classes are alien. Cornwell (1984) shows that health education is only effective if it changes private perceptions, and when self-esteem is low, health education needs to be given in a way that supports and does not further undermine esteem, and which is accessible, as otherwise it will not be effective. Learning is not likely to happen if there are barriers, and a lot of effort went into reducing the 'them and us' lines through sharing, perhaps a cup of tea or experiences about children. Not being judgemental was vitally important, and this is a large issue as cultural codes, which create the barriers, are not held in common. It was through trying to make sense of these classes that a theoretical framework emerged about some of the mechanisms that women developed for coping with long-term unemployment and which were a challenge to work with for the midwives.

THEORY

After the midwives had worked in the area, having taught the classes and seen various patterns of behaviour repeating themselves throughout the estate, a theory began to emerge that there were consistencies that could be identified (Glaser & Strauss 1967). The first was that during the group sessions the topic of conversation would jump about from one thing to another, and rarely was one topic developed fully. The second was that the women kept moving house.

The theory developed was referred to as the 'waterboatman theory', describing the phenomenon of flitting about on the surface, and referring to the observation that this appears to be one way in which economically disadvantaged women cope. In order to survive long-term poverty (Jackson 1982), with its debt and despair, women learn to skate along on the surface like waterboatmen. It is better to develop a means of staying on top, which they appear to do by keeping moving, skittering from subject to subject, in any direction, without the intention of or necessarily getting there but with the realisation that if they stopped to consider, or ponder on problems, they would sink. This explained the difficulty experienced when trying to keep to any definite topic during the sessions.

This was not a reflection of competence on the part of the women, but reflected a way of keeping going, of coping. It was quite disconcerting to be discussing, for example, pain relief in labour, to suddenly have the topic moved to the use of drugs for 'recreational' use, and how their use by partners was having an impact on the women. These diversions were frequently dramatic, often recounted entertainingly, but were also disturbing, both in their content and as diversions. They highlighted the divide between an often naive professional who could concentrate, and the worldly, streetwise group of women living very near a variety of very dangerous edges, who would not concentrate for fear of falling.

The theory was supported through a study of 80 women (Davies 1995) using semistructured questionnaires that looked at social activity, experience of health and family networks. This study was a result of questions that were raised by observations made during the project. One observation was made that women frequently moved house; these moves were mapped as the frequency was extraordinary. The maps made a graphic representation of the theory, as they showed patterns of how the women changed course and kept on the move, without actually moving away. There were five mappings carried out on the estate, each with 16 women's house moving drawn. All the maps show similar patterns of movement (Figure 4.1).

Figure 4.1   *The house moves of 16 women on the estate*

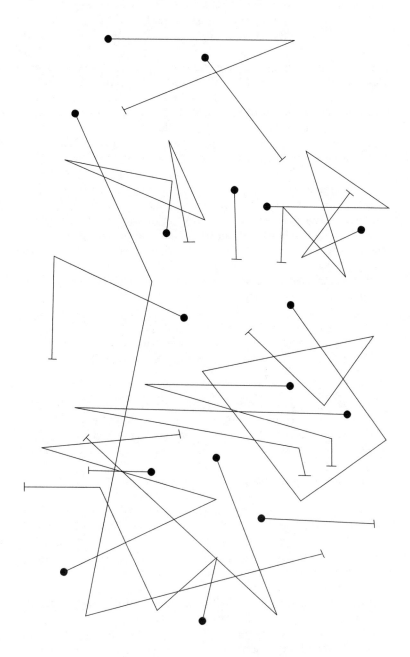

House moving was a common activity on the estate. Housing was blamed for many problems and it was thought that, by moving, there was an escape from these. However, underlying problems relating to debt and poverty could only be alleviated for a period, and even this alleviation stopped when the social security payments for house removal and furniture were stopped, and loans were offered instead. When sought, many of these loans were refused because they were only given if there was evidence that they would be repaid. The fact that the moves were repeated indicates that here was an idiosyncratic response to living and being trapped economically. Sixty-five per cent of the occupants had rent arrears in 1989. The housing department had allowed this situation to arise, and the residents were not rehoused in council property off the estate if they owed money, but the council recognised that moving tenants within the estate could reduce some of the tensions that arose, and consequently house moving was common. Around it arose complex issues of supply and demand, control and coercion, sometimes expressed by vandalism. These were issues that were difficult for the locally based housing department officers to deal with. The midwives worked in close liaison with them: the housing department was in the other half of the semidetached building that housed the neighbourhood centre. There was a multidisciplinary task group in which others, such as teachers and probation officers, worked towards a cohesive approach to care in the community. This group formed a forum for discussing the particular constraints that each group had. There were health issues that provided particular challenges to midwives.

Smoking

Seventy-six per cent of the women in the study smoked. During the classes a 'no smoking' period was achieved. It had to be constantly reinforced and was treated at times with derision, the women simply going outside to smoke. However, they came back, although some tried to light up before the allotted period was over, but the directive approach within an overall non-directive session highlighted smoking as an important issue. There was always a lot of discussion about it. Information about babies being smaller if the women smoked during pregnancy was welcomed as a 'good thing' since most women believed that delivering a smaller baby would be easier. There was always also the tale told of so-and-so who smoked 40 a day and produced a nine pounder, which was presented as proof that the midwives did not know what they were talking about.

The view was often expressed that health workers, including midwives, were inadequate innocents who did not have a clue what they were talking about. They obviously lacked street credibility in the harsh world of the inner city where cigarettes were often cited as the 'only pleasure' there was to be had. Notwithstanding this, however, the message about smoking was reinforced at every contact, often with humour and banter, and the fact that the women continued to attend the group indicated that the ban was not a barrier. It is possible that the tea, the chat and the 'food spot' counteracted the smoking ban. One of the most persistent smokers gave up some time after attending the group; she said it was being told so often about it that made her eventually stop.

Nutrition

Initially, the idea had been to have cooking sessions at the classes, but the kitchen was not safe because there were often children underfoot. Consequently, the midwives brought in food made at home. This was partly to introduce new foods and bring nutrition into the discussion, but it was also important as a social act, reducing the barriers between 'them and us' that prevented views being exchanged and ideas being transmitted. The idea of nettle soup was greeted with horror, but the soup was tasted with interest.

Food is obviously an essential component of health. In the study of 80 women, 53 per cent had not eaten either fruit or vegetables the day before the interview, 37.5 per cent had eaten nothing on the day of the interview and two women had eaten nothing at all the day before the interview. One commented that when she got the shakes she just drank some pop, which made her feel better, along with a cigarette. Two women said that they 'regularly' had a bowel movement only once a fortnight, and eight said it was only once a week; it is difficult for a midwife to stop asking about this even in a research project (Davies 1989).

Self-Esteem

Pregnancy is the ideal time for introducing and developing an awareness of health and the self-esteem that is essential for a positive approach to parenting (Aarvold & Davies 1995). The work that was undertaken in the neighbourhood centre was not only antenatal classes, although these definitely opened the way for some of the women to attend other community development events in the centre. These have evolved, and now there is an active group, organising holidays, children's parties and other activities.

The neighbourhood centre, which was established with the Community Midwifery Care Project and the social services department, had a common philosophy of health promotion through encouraging individual participation. The centre developed, has a local management committee and is now a focus of community development on the estate. With funding support from Save the Children, the work continues under the name of the Community and Family Health Project. Through being involved in the centre, many women have become active in the community and received support from each other, and it has given a focus for activities for the children during the school holidays. Above all, some women have been able to gain self-esteem through this involvement.

Experience of health

A meeting was organised by the health authority and the social services department to discuss health on the estate. Noise was an issue, sleep being frequently disturbed by cars being used for 'joy riding' around the estate. Dogs were another problem, identified as being a health hazard: they would empty the contents of dustbins. A period of free spaying was arranged, and dog sterilisation provided a new angle on family planning.

One of the most important issues that emerged was the perceived effect of violence, and the fear of violence, on wellbeing and the ability to be healthy. The fear of burglary made prisons of people's homes, but what also emerged was that there was often fear within the home.

In the study, the 80 women were asked about their perceptions of health: 75 per cent said that they had health problems. However, only 33 per cent of these had a medical component, 66 per cent related to family, finance, housing and education issues. Of the 25 women who felt that their health was suffering because of family problems, the breakdown of concerns is shown in Table 4.2.

Table 4.2   *Health problems attributed to the family situation*

Problem	No. of women
Violence	7
Alcohol and drugs	5
Child abuse	4
Divorce	1
Daughters' boyfriends	2
Child's death	1
Family pressure	3
Children disturbed	2

Thirty-three of the women studied (41 per cent) had visited their GP during the week of the interview. Given that 66 per cent of the recorded health problems were not medical matters, it would seem that here is evidence of yet another divide, or gap, between what this group of women perceive as their problems and the ability of those to whom they turn to do anything about them. That expressed health needs cannot be matched with conventional medical provision may be universal to those with low income.

What was clear was that health was perceived as not only relating to medical issues, although the women turned to their GPs. This is a dilemma, as it is not within the GPs' powers to address some of the issues on which they are consulted, these being social and economic rather than medical issues. As the steps towards primary care (NHS Executive 1996) take place, the question must be raised of whether conventional primary health care is the appropriate way in which to address the issue of health care provision for groups of low-income women, or whether having some-thing that is community- rather than clinic- or practice-based, where there are facilities for active self-development rather than passive treat-ment, would address the challenge of low-income women more effectively.

CULTURE

There are cultural and lifestyle issues that clearly relate directly to health, both physical and mental. Only 35 per cent of the women were married; another 37.5 per cent were single and cohabiting. In some cases, however, the man and woman claimed state benefit separately as a way of maximising their income. A number of women said that this gave them an economic security that was absent in joint claims, which were often out of their hands.

This separate claiming could put a strain on relationships within the partnership as there was always the fear of being caught or of someone reporting it. This kind of information was always a source of tension within the community, which could erupt if there were any quarrels between neighbours or even within the families themselves. It undermined any sense of family cohesion, and the poor role model for the young boys of fathers who were neither at home nor economically connected reinforced long-term dependence on welfare (Davies 1992).

The women in the study lived very locally, often seeing their mothers daily, and 80 per cent seeing them at least once a week. The men appeared to be marginal to the daily activities of the children, even though they were not in employment. The most frequent female activity reported was collecting children from school, which 69 per cent did at least once a day. Only 14 per cent of the women had any work, that being all part-time, short-term work. One woman cleaned the Magistrates' Court. It gave her a sense of 'justice' that she was working illegally at the court, which she saw as a tool of 'them'. The work was illegal in that she was also claiming benefit, a fairly common activity that was another source of possible community disruption if knowledge about it was used as a weapon in disputes. The men on the estate had similarly low employment rates.

ECONOMIC DIVIDE

A person living on welfare in Britain might be materially better off than someone living in the Third World, but the economic divide within the country is increasing. During the period of the study, this growing division became visible with the removal of single payments being available for large items that people periodically needed and a loan system introduced. This reduced standards of living as these loans were often refused because of the inability to repay them. Consequently, the goods for which pervasive advertising creates a need were increasingly difficult to obtain. Houses became markedly shabbier in the aftermath of this. The alienation created by the inability to buy what is readily available, but which is urged on all as being essential, seemed to increase the illegal pursuit of these goods. The reappearance in the estate of bedding plants from an adjacent roundabout was a fairly benign manifestation of economic restructuring. There were a considerable number less benignly occupied, and children below the age of legal responsibility were often commandeered into illegal activities. Raising a family in a neighbourhood where this kind of activity was common was very hard for those who wished to eschew this approach.

Long-term unemployment and dependence on welfare are increasingly becoming major political issues as demographic changes in the economic make-up of Britain occur (*Independent* 1993). With the aging population and high unemployment rates, costs are increasing and political reactions about how welfare should be managed increasingly reflect the divide between 'them and us'. At one end of the spectrum are highly paid executives working within private and public enterprises; at the other end are the long-term unemployed on benefits.

CHALLENGES FOR MIDWIVES

When evaluating the Community Midwifery Care Project, Evans (1987) remarked that a number of the women had commented that the midwives were 'one of us'. From a number of standpoints, not least economic, this was not true, although obviously in other areas there were commonalities, in particular the shared experience of children. That some women felt this relationship shows that it is possible for midwives to meet the challenge of being 'with woman'. This does, however, require an effort to break down some of the barriers that professionals sometimes choose to erect as a means of proclaiming their separate status. This is achievable in a variety of ways, one being through providing very local, women-centred care designed to meet the specific needs of a particular group (Department of Health 1993).

One essential aspect of midwifery is accepting the social integrity of individual women and working to establish ways in which this is upheld. This applies to working with women of any cultural background different from the midwife's and demands a need for self-awareness and reflection about the cultural component of being a midwife. If a woman is unsure of her own self-worth, it is doubly important that midwives help her build it. Birth is a crucial time for women, and midwives have a great responsibility, and challenge, to guide women into motherhood in such a way as to give them worth – for 'them' individually, and for 'us' collectively.

Using a groupwork approach to parentcraft classes created a forum in which midwives helped women's confidence to grow, and where issues of childcare were raised. These included such topics as the importance of play and positive communication with children. If women are to be supported as they become mothers, it is essential to accept who they are in the first instance.

Much of this work is very low key, but this is a time when 'being with' a woman can affect her psychic development, alter the direction of her life and affect her parenting. It is increasingly important for the children of tomorrow's rapidly changing world to have good parenting today. If, by being 'with woman', midwives can reduce the gaps between 'them and us', not in the economic sphere but by enabling women to have self-worth, they will be meeting a great challenge. Midwifery is a challenge in itself, but there is the even greater challenge of showing that in a society where childcare is becoming a political issue, midwives have a crucial role to play in how tomorrow's children are reared. How women experience the 'rite of passage' of becoming a mother can affect that, and it is the midwives' role to be with them during this crucial transition to make it women-centred. It is a challenge to raise an awareness of just how crucial this time is if there is to be a change 'Towards a Healthy Nation' (Royal College of Midwives 1992).

REFERENCES

Aarvold J, Davies J 1995 Community Maternity Care. In Heyman B (ed.) *Researching Health Care* London: Chapman & Hall

Child Poverty Action Group 1996 *Poverty: The facts*. London: CPAG

Cornwell J 1984 *Hard Earned Lives: Accounts of health and illness from East London*. London: Tavistock

Davies J 1989 Tangled Webs: Family networks and activity examined in one inner city area. MSc dissertation, Faculty of Social Sciences, Northumbria University

Davies J 1995 A Study of family networks. In Reed J, Proctor S (eds) *Practitioner Research in Health Care*. London: Chapman & Hall

Davies Jon G (ed.) 1992 *From Household to Family to Individualism. The family: Is it just another lifestyle choice?* London: IEA Health and Welfare Unit

DHSS 1980a *House of Commons Social Services Committee Report on Perinatal and Neonatal Mortality (the Short Report)*. London: HMSO

DHSS 1980b *Inequalities in health: Report of a Research Working Group (the Black Report)*. London: HMSO

DHSS 1986 *Neighbourhood Nursing – A Focus for Care (the Cumberlege Report)*. London: HMSO

Department of Health 1993 *Changing Childbirth. A Report of the Expert Maternity Group*. London: HMSO

Downe S 1991 The price of motherhood. *Nursing Times* **87**(10):13–15

Evans F 1987 An Evaluation Report. Newcastle Community Midwifery Care Project, Newcastle Health Authority

Glaser BG, Strauss AL 1967 *The Discovery of Grounded Theory*. Chicago: Aldine

Independent 1993 Lone parents are target for benefit cuts. 10/11/93

International Confederation of Midwives (ICM) 1993 Midwives Hear the Heartbeat of the Future. Proceedings of 23rd International Confederation of Midwives, Vancouver, Canada, 10–14 May

Jackson B 1982 *How the Poorest Live, New Society Social Studies Reader*, 2nd edn. London: New Society

NHS Executive 1996 *Primary Care: The future*. London: HMSO

Royal College of Midwives (RCM) *Towards a Healthy Nation* 1992 London: RCM

CHAPTER FIVE

Midwifery care and female genital mutilation

Joanna Hindley and Sarah Montagu

Female genital mutilation (FGM) is a traditional practice thousands of years old that affects an estimated 80 000 000 women and young girls world wide. Until recently, it was referred to by the euphemism 'female circumcision', which underplayed its life-altering and life-threatening sequelae by allowing confusion with male circumcision. Its effects on a woman's sexuality and her experience of pregnancy and childbirth are particularly profound and therefore pose a challenge to the midwives who will care for her.

FGM most commonly occurs in certain parts of Africa and the Middle East. In some communities, as many as 98 per cent of women and girls will be mutilated. However, the increased mobility of world populations due to poverty, war and famine means that FGM will also be encountered in countries in the developed world. In the UK, the Prohibition of Female Circumcision Act, passed in 1985, made the practice illegal; nevertheless, it is still practised secretly in Britain (Black & Debelle 1995).

Several factors, such as the breakdown of traditional societies, advancement in women's status and increased international recognition of women's and children's rights, for example in the UN Convention on the Rights of the Child (1989), have brought about a more open discussion of FGM. This has led to its widespread condemnation as a practice and to campaigns for its eradication. The World Health Organization has taken up the cause and drawn up specific recommendations for action (WHO 1995).

Midwives caring for genitally mutilated women will be challenged to reassess their expectations and practice that have been based on the Western norm of uncircumcised genitalia. They will also need to address issues of racism, ethnocentrism and the status of women in general.

WHAT IS FGM?

It is assumed you are already aware of the anatomy of normal, intact female genitalia and their role and function in female sexuality, pregnancy and childbirth. In order to provide effective care for women who have been genitally mutilated, you will also need to be aware of the forms of FGM and the anatomical structures affected by each.

Figure 5.1 *Diagrams of intact and infibulated vulva (reproduced with the permission of Minority Rights Group International)*

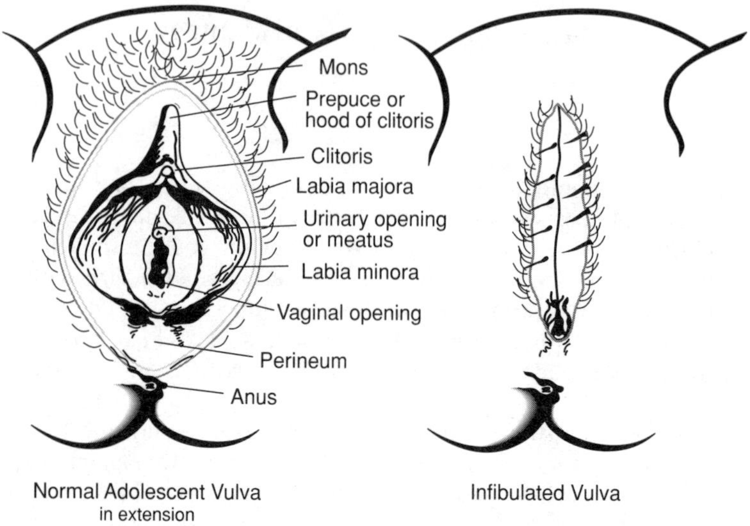
Mons
Prepuce or
hood of clitoris
Clitoris
Labia majora
Urinary opening
or meatus
Labia minora
Vaginal opening
Perineum
Anus
Normal Adolescent Vulva
in extension
Infibulated Vulva

There are three main forms of female genital mutilation (Figure 5.1):

1. Circumcision – separation/removal of the prepuce (hood of the clitoris).
2. Excision – removal of the clitoris, or removal of the clitoris and all or part of the labia minora.
3. Infibulation or 'pharaonic' circumcision – excision, including removal of the labia majora and suturing together of the raw sides, leaving one very small opening (Dorkenoo & Elworthy 1992).

CULTURAL AND ETHNIC GROUPS WITHIN WHICH FGM IS PRACTISED

In Africa, the belt in which mutilation is commonly practised stretches from Senegal in the west to Egypt in the north east and Tanzania in the south east.

The numbers of women and girls affected may be viewed as percentages of the national population. For example, in Somalia virtually 100 per cent are affected, and in the Sudan, Ethiopia, Mali and Sierra Leone, 90 per cent (Dorkenoo & Elworthy 1992). However, the absolute numbers should not be overlooked; for example, although only 50 per cent of women in Nigeria are affected, as Nigeria is the most populated African country, this accounts for one third of the total estimate of 60–80 million.

Infibulation, the severest form of genital mutilation, is most common in Mali, Sudan, Ethiopia, Somalia and Northern Nigeria. However, FGM is not exclusively an African practice. Excision takes place in the Middle Eastern countries of Oman, South Yemen and the United Arab Emirates (UAE). Circumcision is practised by the Muslim populations of Indonesia and Malaysia, and by some Muslim groups in India, Pakistan and East Africa (Dorkenoo & Elworthy 1992).

FGM is not unknown in the West. Clitoridectomies were performed in the nineteenth and even twentieth centuries by gynaecologists to control allegedly deviant sexual behaviours such as masturbation, hysteria and other so-called female disorders (Passmore-Sanderson 1981).

INTERNATIONAL CONVENTIONS AND NATIONAL LEGISLATION PROHIBITING FGM

In September 1990 the United Nations Convention on the Rights of the Child came into force, bringing FGM into the sphere of International Human Rights Legislation. Article 24(3) of this Convention states that 'States Parties shall take effective and appropriate measures with a view to abolishing traditional practices prejudicial to the health of children'.

Legislation prohibiting infibulation exists in many African countries, including Sudan, Egypt and Burkina Faso. The Inter-Africa Committee, a non-governmental organisation, is co-ordinating 'grass-roots' activities against FGM from its headquarters in Addis Ababa, Ethiopia. Several religious leaders in Africa have made statements clarifying the position regarding FGM in Islam and Christianity, as it has been mistakenly assumed to be a religious requirement (Al Naggar & Assad 1985).

Many European countries have enacted specific legislation banning FGM, for example Sweden, the Netherlands, Belgium and the UK, where the Prohibition of Female Circumcision Act has been in force since 1985 (Dorkenoo & Elworthy 1992).

The UK's Children Act 1989, Section 47(1) empowers local authorities to investigate if they have 'reasonable cause to suspect that a child who lives, or is found, in their area is suffering, or is likely to suffer, significant harm'. Under the Act, as a last resort, a Prohibitive Steps Order can be made to prevent parents from removing a child in order to carry out a mutilation abroad, or a Care Supervision Order can ultimately be sought, if there is no better way of protecting a child considered to be at risk of genital mutilation (Hedley & Dorkenoo 1992).

As part of the World Health Organization's efforts to abolish the practice, a multidisciplinary meeting for delegates from UN countries was held in Geneva in July 1995. Its aims were to define the different types of FGM, to assess the impact of such procedures on women's health, to identify areas for further research and to draw up specific recommendations for action (WHO 1995).

REVIEW OF THE LITERATURE

The existing literature on female genital mutilation has done much to bring the issues involved into the public arena and to carry forward the campaign to eradicate harmful traditional practices.

Historically, the campaign against FGM has been clouded by issues of colonialism and attempts to represent FGM as a legitimate cultural practice both within Africa and among emigrant groups (Walker & Parmar 1993). One of the most important developments has therefore been the involvement of African women, who are able to relate the issue of FGM to the status of women in Africa in general and to campaign from within the African community against its continuation (El Saadawi 1980; Thiam 1986). It is particularly important for anyone involved in working with the communities that most commonly practise FGM to read these and similar books in order to understand the relevant issues of culture, tradition and women's and children's rights.

The Pulitzer Prize-winning novelist Alice Walker has written a novel that centres on the theme of FGM and the devastating effect it has on women's lives (Walker 1992). She has also collaborated in the production of a documentary film that has shown both the strength of the traditional forces which would maintain the practice and the progress of the movement towards its eradication (Walker & Parmar 1993). However, although there is general material as well as specific guidelines for workers in the community who may be involved in education or child protection work (Hedley & Dorkenoo 1992), there is little practical advice for health care workers who are faced with giving physical and psychological care to mutilated women.

IMPLICATIONS OF FGM FOR WOMEN

FGM affects every aspect of a woman's sexual and reproductive life. A woman who has undergone mutilation may well have a damaged sense of herself as a woman, particularly if the practice of FGM conflicts with her own beliefs and values. The physical and psychological pain that persists after FGM can completely destroy a woman's sexual pleasure (El Saadawi 1980).

There are damaging consequences from all forms of FGM but the most severe are associated with infibulation. In some cases, excessive vulval scarring leads to anal or even urethral intercourse taking place. The trauma resulting from intercourse increases the likelihood of infection and the transmission of the human immunodeficiency virus. Repeated infections can lead to internal inflammation and scarring, diminishing the chances of conception and at worst resulting in infertility.

In pregnancy, there are likely to be physical problems resulting from the mutilation, including a greater than normal risk of urinary tract infections and vaginal thrush. Certain of the minor disorders of pregnancy, such as frequency of micturition, increased leucorrhoea and pelvic congestion, will be exacerbated.

Fear and anxiety about possible reactions from health professionals may lead to a reluctance to attend for antenatal care, especially if the woman feels she might be internally examined. She will also be likely to feel apprehensive about the delivery itself and how it will be managed.

Labour and delivery present a number of difficulties for the woman, primarily because the sensations and pain may recall her vulnerability at the initial mutilation and the trauma associated with it. She may find herself once again immobilised, flat on her back, exposed and defenceless, feeling her genitals being touched and viewed by strangers. She may not only have to deal with her own feelings, but may also have to cope with the reactions of midwives unprepared for caring for someone affected by FGM, as the following case history illustrates.

A young Somali woman living in Cardiff was admitted to the local maternity unit in suspected early labour. 'I was having my first baby. The midwife wanted to examine me to see if I was really in labour or not. She asked me to pull my dress up and part my legs so that she could do this. An expression of horror came over her face when she saw me and she rushed off without saying anything. I felt so afraid and alone. The next thing I knew there were five or six people in white coats all looking at me. I didn't understand what they were saying to each other. The pains were getting worse and nobody was helping me'.

In some cases, it has been found that certain forms of pain relief, for example epidural anaesthesia, are less effective. The pain of mutilation is restimulated and is difficult to alleviate by any of the usual means. Due to health professionals' lack of familiarity with FGM, the woman may find herself subjected to inappropriate interventions and the involvement of greater numbers of midwifery and medical staff than is necessary. The delivery itself will be distressing and painful because it necessitates the stretching and incision of the tough scar tissue of infibulation. Suturing afterwards may pose further problems for the woman, since if she wishes to be reinfibulated, as some women do, she may meet with opposition if the midwife is aware that this would, in effect, contravene the terms of the Prohibition of Female Circumcision Act 1985.

In the postnatal period, the healing process of the sutured areas may be prolonged due to the impaired regenerative capacity of scar tissue. An anterior episiotomy is likely to be very painful, particularly on passing urine, since it involves densely innervated tissue. Should a woman be rein-fibulated, the passage of lochia and postdelivery diuresis will be impaired and will predispose her to infection.

CHALLENGES OF FGM FOR MIDWIFERY PRACTICE

The majority of midwives practising in the developed world have not come across FGM and are not prepared for providing care for a woman affected by it. FGM is not covered within the curricula of most programmes of midwifery education and training. Indeed, in most cases, guidelines for good practice and specific provision have not been developed. Standard midwifery textbooks (e.g. Bennett & Brown 1993; Silverton 1993) make either very brief or no mention of the topic. So, as the following case history indicates, seeing a mutilated woman for the first time can cause appalled confusion.

> A student midwife in a Birmingham maternity unit remembers her shock reaction at seeing the vulva of an infibulated woman and her mystification as to what could have possibly caused this. 'I had never seen anything like it before. There was just nothing there; just skin stretching across where the vulva should have been. I thought she must have had some sort of car accident or something! I went and asked for help but the unit was very busy that day and there was nobody available to help me. I was left to get on as best I could. Looking back on it I think that nobody knew what to do.'

Antenatal care

The main challenges for midwives are to provide sensitive antenatal care, specific preparation for labour and delivery, and appropriate psychological care and counselling. The failure to provide these often leads to unnecessary interventions in labour and delivery, for example bilateral episiotomies or even caesarean sections, as staff are not aware of the more appropriate modes of care.

Many of the obstetric difficulties that can arise when caring for a woman affected by FGM can be obviated by good antenatal preparation and appropriate midwifery care that facilitate the progress of normal labour.

At the booking interview, the midwife needs to be alert to the possibility that women from particular ethnic groups are likely to have undergone genital mutilation. In order to elicit this information, she might ask whether the woman 'has had any special operation when she was young' or whether she has 'been cut'.

Interpreters should be available to translate for women whose first language is not English. Ideally, there should be specific provision for women affected by FGM in the form of a community antenatal clinic catering for their particular needs.

Northwick Park Hospital in Harrow, north London, has set up a specialist clinic offering antenatal care as well as counselling for women with FGM who may wish to undergo deinfibulation in preparation for labour and delivery. They offer deinfibulation with reconstruction of the vulva as far as is possible. This is performed in the second trimester, usually under a general anaesthetic.

In areas where a specific clinic like this is not available, continuity of carer is especially important so that a woman with FGM may build up a trusting relationship with a midwife who is familiar with her particular needs, and can therefore offer sensitive and appropriate care. The midwife can also mobilise other agencies, for example specialist counsellors, and arrange referral for deinfibulation if appropriate.

Guidelines for management of labour and delivery should be discussed with the woman and her partner and with other members of the obstetric and midwifery team, and agreed in advance. An interpreter should be present if required. The midwife plays an important role in ensuring that the woman has access to all the information relevant to her care so that she can make informed decisions.

The midwife should be aware that there is an increased risk of infection in the antenatal period for women who have been infibulated and should therefore give advice on ways of minimising this risk. If infection is suspected, diagnosis may be made more difficult if a high vaginal swab is unobtainable. Treatment may also be complicated by the fact that administration of medication per vaginam may be impossible.

Labour and delivery

The most important contribution the midwife can make to the care of the mutilated woman is to implement true midwifery care, in the sense of being 'with woman'. In no area is this more important than in labour and delivery. If the issues raised by genital mutilation have, for whatever reason, not been addressed during the antenatal period, they must now be confronted.

It may be difficult or impossible to perform vaginal examinations, both for physical reasons and because this may be culturally unacceptable to the woman. This may hinder both the diagnosis of labour and the assessment of its progress. Emphasis may rather be placed on observation of external signs, such as uterine activity and the length, strength and frequency of contractions, or even more subtle indications, such as the woman's behaviour. Where infibulation is present, recourse to rectal examination may be made to assess cervical dilatation.

Monitoring of fetal condition may be carried out by intermittent auscultation. If continuous electronic fetal monitoring is considered necessary, it may be practical only to monitor externally where infibulation makes application of a fetal scalp electrode impossible. Fetal blood sampling and use of an intrauterine pressure catheter will likewise be precluded.

The midwife must assess the woman's need for pain relief and help her to decide what is most appropriate by considering all options available, including non-pharmacological forms of pain relief. The midwife will need to bear in mind that the psychological components of the experience of pain will be particularly strong for the woman who has been genitally mutilated, and she may need to use some of the counselling techniques described by Adamson (1992). It has already been noted, for example, that the pain relief afforded by epidural anaesthesia may be less effective. Administration of a pudendal block, if required, will be complicated by the presence of infibulation, which can so distort the vulval anatomy that it is impossible to locate the pudendal nerve.

Urinary catheterisation may be difficult, if not impossible, to perform where mutilation has altered the normal anatomy. The midwife therefore needs to be particularly careful to ensure that the woman empties her bladder regularly. Other interventions, such as artificial rupture of membranes or prostaglandin induction of labour, may also prove very difficult.

Where infibulation is present, a medial anterior episiotomy will be necessary to expedite delivery. There is some debate over when this is best performed, but it is usually recommended that it be performed as the baby's head begins to crown so that blood loss may be kept to a minimum. Whether or not infibulation is present, the scarred vulval tissue may be more fragile and prone to tear. The episiotomy must be made carefully, to prevent further damage to the area, particularly the urethra.

Repair: the choices

Repair of an episiotomy or a tear will involve decisions about the extent of repair and reconstruction of the vulva. Simply to suture together the two sides of the incision is, in effect, to reinfibulate the woman, which is illegal under the Prohibition of Female Circumcision Act 1985. Midwifery and obstetric staff may be confronted by the request to perform this type of repair and need to be aware of the relevant legislation. The repair must involve recreating a vulval opening by stitching over each of the raw sides so they do not appose. The suture material of choice is a polyglycolic acid suture (such as Dexon or Vicryl) as this causes less inflammation and is less likely to fall out before the healing process is sufficiently far advanced for the sides of the vulva not to reappose.

The puerperium

In the postnatal period, vulval as well as possibly perineal healing needs to be observed, and the woman should be advised about hygiene, good nutrition and the use of pelvic floor exercises to promote healing. However, the midwife's role in providing psychological and educational support is as important as it is in giving physical care. Both the woman and her partner will need to come to terms with her body image, which has been altered yet again. They may be offered referral to a specialist counsellor (Adamson 1992).

The midwife should discuss with the women and her partner the appropriate timing for resumption of sexual relations. This will depend on the mode of delivery and the stage of healing of the perineal tissue. She should raise the issue of family planning and should present information on the various methods available, enabling the couple to make an informed choice appropriate to their needs, preferences and cultural requirements.

Child protection issues

If the child is a girl, the need to protect her against being genitally mutilated should be addressed. It is not too early to mobilise counselling and support to avert potential mutilation. This may need to involve the extended family too, as older family members may put considerable pressure on the new parents to have them conform to tradition (Hedley & Dorkenoo 1992).

Hedley and Dorkenoo (1992) propose a workable system of child protection. They advocate the use of a specialist trained advisor (STA) appointed by the local authority social services department, who may be a midwife, health visitor, social worker or other well-placed professional. The STA will advise, support, counsel and work together with the family to protect the child (Adamson 1992).

Although social services departments have the primary responsibility for ensuring implementation of the child protection system, midwives should make sure that they are included in STA training programmes.

It is estimated that as many as 10 000 girl children in the UK are at risk of genital mutilation (de Silva 1994). Figure 5.2 outlines a proposed child protection system.

Figure 5.2   *A child protection system for FGM (reproduced with the permission of FORWARD UK)*

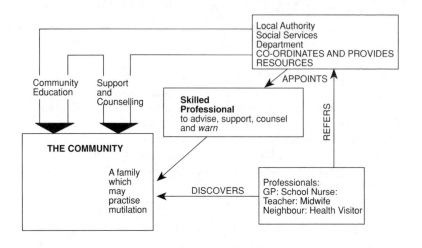

RECOMMENDATIONS FOR MIDWIFERY PRACTICE

The subject of FGM needs to be adequately covered both within programmes of midwifery education and in standard midwifery textbooks. This would ensure that midwives entering the profession are sufficiently aware of its implications for midwifery practice.

In-service training and study days should be provided for midwives who are already in practice, and the topic of FGM should be included in refresher courses and midwifery update programmes. Guidelines for good practice should be developed and disseminated as widely as possible.

All midwifery units, and certainly those used by a large number of women affected by FGM, should consider making specific provision of care. This should include specially trained midwives, specific antenatal clinics, the availability of interpreters, the provision of specially trained counsellors and the development of channels for referral to specialist centres, for example for deinfibulation.

Links with social services and education departments should be developed in order to co-ordinate action related to child protection and the prevention of FGM.

Practice check

The UKCC Code of Professional Conduct (1993, Clause 7) urges each registered nurse, midwife and health visitor to:

> recognise and respect the uniqueness and dignity of each patient and client, and respond to their need for care, irrespective of their ethnic origin, religious beliefs, personal attributes, the nature of their health problems or any other factor.

With this in mind, ask yourself the following questions:

- How will I feel if confronted with a woman presenting in labour who has undergone FGM?
- Do I feel comfortable with issues relating to sexuality? Do these feelings affect how I might behave towards a woman who has been genitally mutilated?
- What is my attitude towards traditional practices that are prejudicial to health and wellbeing? Is this attitude affected by racism?
- Is my ability to speak out against FGM hindered by a fear of being called racist?
- What provisions are there in my local area for women affected by FGM?
- How shall I go about protecting a young girl when I think she might be at risk of genital mutilation?
- How shall I ensure the privacy of a woman in my care who has been genitally mutilated?
- What am I doing to further my own and others' understanding and awareness of the issues surrounding FGM?

SUMMARY

This chapter has highlighted the main challenges confronting midwives when caring for women who have been genitally mutilated. Perhaps the greatest challenge is for the midwife to develop confidence in her own midwifery skills and to feel that she is competent to deliver physical and psychological care to meet these women's needs despite the serious effects of the mutilation they have suffered.

By encouraging readers to think about their own attitudes, practice and the implications in the context of Clause 7 of the UKCC Code of Professional Conduct, the chapter's intention has been to encourage and enable midwives to prepare themselves to care for women who have been genitally mutilated. It may also be used to form the basis for developing standards of care at a local level.

ACKNOWLEDGEMENTS

Thanks are due to Efua Dorkenoo and FORWARD International, to Comfort Ottah, and to Mary McCaffery and Northwick Park Hospital.

REFERENCES

Adamson F 1992 *Female Genital Mutilation: A counselling guide for professionals.* London: FORWARD

Al Naggar A, Assad M 1985 *Female Circumcision and Religion.* Cairo: Family Planning Association, Maternal and Child Health Programme

Bennett V, Brown L (eds) 1993 *Myles Textbook for Midwives,* 12th edn. Edinburgh: Churchill Livingstone

Black JA, Debelle GD 1995 Female genital mutilation in Britain. *British Medical Journal* **310**:1590–4

de Silva S 1994 *Women in medicine* September:16–21

Dorkenoo E, Elworthy S 1992 *Female Genital Mutilation: Proposals for change.* London: Minority Rights Group

El Saadawi N 1980 *The Hidden Face of Eve.* London: Zed Press

Hedley R, Dorkenoo E 1992 *Child Protection and Female Genital Mutilation.* London: FORWARD

Passmore-Sanderson L 1981 *Against the Mutilation of Women: The struggle to end unnecessary suffering.* London: Ithaca Press

Silverton L 1993 *The Art and Science of Midwifery.* London: Prentice Hall

Thiam A 1986 *African Women Speak out: Feminism and oppression in Black Africa.* London: Pluto Press

Walker A 1992 *Possessing the Secret of Joy.* London: Jonathan Cape

Walker A, Parmar P 1993 *Warrior Marks.* London: Jonathan Cape

World Health Organization (WHO) 1995 *WHO Continues its Battle Against Female Genital Mutilation.* Geneva: WHO

FURTHER INFORMATION

Books

Dorkenoo E 1992 *Tradition! Tradition!* London: FORWARD

El Dareer A 1982 *Woman, Why Do You Weep?* London: Zed Press

Koso-Thomas O 1987 *The Circumcision of Women: A strategy for eradication.* London: Zed Press

Films and videos

Another Form of Abuse 1992 London: FORWARD

Cruel Ritual 1991 London: BBC Enterprises

Warrior Marks 1993 London: Channel Four

USEFUL ADDRESSES

FORWARD International (Foundation for Women's Health, Research &
Development)
Africa Centre
38 King Street
London WC2E 8JT   Tel: 0171–379 6889

IAC (Inter-African Committee on Traditional Practices Affecting the Health of
Women and Children)
147 Rue de Lausanne
CH-1202
Geneva
Switzerland

Northwick Park Hospital Department of Obstetrics & Gynaecology
Watford Road
Harrow
Middlesex HA1 3UJ   Tel: 0181–869 2880

CHAPTER SIX

Hearing impairment and midwifery care

Jennifer Kelsall

As the key professional, companion and communicator for women during pregnancy and the puerperium, the midwife will sometimes be faced with additional challenges. Where a woman has impaired hearing, or where her baby is born deaf, particular strategies will be needed to ensure that both mother and infant receive the care they deserve. Within this context, midwives' responsibilities cover two distinct areas. First, they must be aware of the possibility of inherited or acquired deafness and ensure that no baby who may be at risk is denied early screening. Second, deaf parents presenting for maternity care must have their deafness and preferred communication method considered and recorded so that such care can be tailored to meet their needs (Kelsall *et al.* 1992).

HEARING IMPAIRMENT IN THE NEWBORN

Congenital deafness: asking the right questions

Many of the implications of caring for the parents of a deaf baby will be similar to those of caring for parents whose baby has any congenital handicap (see Chapter 3). This chapter will concern itself with the specifics of hearing impairment.

Midwives should be aware that 1 in 1000 babies is born with a congenital hearing loss and even today these babies are not always identified. During the antenatal period, midwives are in a key position to identify those babies likely to be born with deficient hearing.

At the antenatal booking interview, *all* women receiving antenatal care should be asked the same simple questions about familial hearing problems. If any member of either parent's family has any history of deafness in childhood – particularly where a hearing aid was employed – there is an increased likelihood of hearing impairment being inherited. If the deafness is known to have been acquired through infection or injury, then it will not be inherited. If the cause of deafness is, however, in any way uncertain or unknown, early screening of the newborn infant should be arranged.

Knowing what questions to ask during pregnancy and ensuring that hearing tests occur after birth will not happen automatically unless specific policies are introduced wherever women receive antenatal care. Antenatal booking forms and computerised booking checklists should always include relevant questions about hearing. Information about the importance of implementing this should be included in all midwifery education programmes.

If a fetus is diagnosed as being at risk of congenital deafness, parents should be given appropriate information and support. Explanation of the available hearing tests involved for their baby, support services and counselling should be available from paediatricians, paediatric audiologists or genetic counsellors. After the birth, it is most important that midwives, paediatricians, GPs and health visitors are all aware that early hearing tests are to be carried out. Good communication links between health professionals are essential if a problem is to be identified. Each unit should have a recognised protocol for arranging early hearing tests, together with suitable counselling and support for parents.

Acquired deafness

Not all hearing impairment in infants is inherited. Some babies can be born deaf or are at risk of becoming deaf soon after birth for other reasons. For example (Robertson 1986):

- babies born to mothers who have had rubella in the first trimester of pregnancy (this is less common in developed countries today with the implementation of mass screening and vaccination programmes);
- babies with any craniofacial abnormalities;
- babies with Down syndrome;
- babies with known brain damage;
- babies who have had hyperbilirubinaemia, that is, if the serum bilirubin exceeds the levels indicated in Table 6.1, the risk being greatest with small babies;
- babies with possible aminoglycoside toxicity, that is, as a result of receiving gentamycin/netilmycin therapy or other antibiotics if administered in very large doses;
- babies in whom cytomegalovirus infection has been detected;
- babies with other viral infections – TORCH screen for toxoplasmosis, rubella, cytomegalovirus, herpes and other viruses;
- all babies who have been nursed in incubators in neonatal units for prolonged periods, as high levels of noise within incubators can affect immature hearing.

Early hearing tests should be arranged for babies to whom any of the above applies, as they will be at increased risk of possible hearing damage.

Table 6.1 *Serum bilirubin levels denoting hyperbilirubinaemia*

Gestation in weeks	Serum bilirubin (μmol/l)
28	180
30	210
32	250
34	270
36	290
38	350

Appreciating the impact of infant deafness on parents

While identifying babies who may be at risk of impaired hearing, it is important to be sensitive to the effect that the discovery of potential deafness might have on the parents. Not surprisingly, parents who have hearing loss themselves, even where this is profound, know that they will cope with the problems of deafness in their child. They are likely to mother the baby, love him and communicate with him. Their baby may often learn sign language as its first language. Hearing parents, for whom the soundless world is unmapped territory, are likely to find the news much more difficult to deal with. From the perspective of those who take their own hearing for granted, deafness is a disability that is not understood. As such, parents are likely to perceive it as an enormous handicap and may lack confidence in their ability ever to communicate with their baby.

Parents should be reassured, in the first instance, that they will be able to help their baby. Any baby thrives where it is loved, and the deaf baby must still be loved, cuddled and played with in the same way as any hearing child. The parents must be encouraged to talk to the baby in exactly the same way as they would a hearing child, and the importance of holding the baby close so that he or she can see the parent's face should be explained. In order to learn about communicating and how to lip-read, the hearing-impaired child needs to see the facial expression and speech as it occurs on the lips. Additionally, he or she needs to see language on the lips of the speaker occurring naturally, rather in an artificial, noun-only format. Only after understanding language does language itself develop. This is apparent when one considers any toddler, obviously understanding what is being said but as yet only uttering a few words. That child's understanding of language would be greatly inhibited if he or she had only heard nouns out of context. The same is true of the deaf child, who needs exposure to ordinary conversation but with the obvious visual element being emphasised.

As the child begins to babble, as all babies do, a hearing aid will amplify any hearing the baby may have and enable it possibly to hear its own voice and begin to make some sense of any noises it hears. Where a baby is profoundly deaf, the parents may wish and should be encouraged to learn sign language and use this alongside speech in order to communicate with the child. Expert guidance from a speech therapist will be needed at this stage.

The midwife must support the parents in the care of their child and understand their anxieties, at the same time emphasising that love, normal mothering, baby talk and conversation are just as important for the deaf baby as for the hearing child. In this way, parents can be helped to provide the best foundation for developing whatever communication method their child's hearing impairment warrants.

MATERNITY CARE FOR HEARING-IMPAIRED PARENTS

The midwife is in a position of particular closeness to women and, where continuity of care is properly organised, has several months in which to develop a supportive and trusting relationship as well as being 'with woman' while she is in labour. Kirkham (1986) sees the midwife as being 'the supporter and sometimes therefore the defender of the woman she cares for in labour' and adds, 'but to achieve this we must really concentrate on the woman and her needs'. The positive influence of support during labour itself has been established (McNiven & Hodnett 1992; Hodnett 1994), as has the identification of isolation in the postnatal period as a risk factor for depression (Holden 1990). Yet many deaf mothers experience frustration and loneliness during pregnancy, birth and the puerperium (Jackson 1990). Postnatal discussion with one woman in Manchester showed up the inadequacies of well-intentioned care. This stimulated an initiative to improve the situation and the development of the Maternity Care for the Deaf project in Manchester. If properly informed, midwives can play a pivotal role in the provision of maternity care that is individually suited to parents with hearing problems (Kelsall 1993; Nolan 1994). Unless midwives rise to this challenge, parents with hearing impairment receive inadequate and inappropriate care.

Establishing a rapport with the woman with hearing impairment

Deafness means isolation in the hearing world (Jackson 1990). Conversation is either missing, muffled or misunderstood. General understanding is difficult, and communication – an essential in all maternity care – is minimal. There is an additional stigma attached to deafness that sometimes makes individuals shy about admitting it. Socially, they may be subjected to intolerance, insensitive shouting or joking.

Deafness varies in degree, and each person's impairment is individual. People compensate by wearing hearing aids, lip-reading and using body language or sign language. At the first contact with a deaf woman, the midwife should establish:

- the cause of deafness if it is known, in particular whether it is congenital or acquired;
- the extent of the deafness;
- how the deaf woman chooses to communicate.

The midwife should be aware that there may be mutual difficulties in understanding, and that the woman and the midwife are partners who must strive to overcome them.

It would be wrong to assume that hearing aids will replace lost hearing. They do not – but they do accentuate any residual hearing. Unfortunately, they also augment background noise, and this should be remembered in a noisy hospital setting. Similarly, lip-reading is far from easy, and 60 per cent of any understanding is gleaned by guesswork. The language of pregnancy and childbirth is new, and previously unseen on the lips, so it is likely that misunderstandings will occur.

Visibility is essential for lip-reading. The speaker's mouth must be in good light and he or she must face the deaf person. Those who use sign language must have a qualified interpreter with them, particularly during clinic visits and while they are in labour. The word 'qualified' is used advisedly. If someone with minimal sign language skills is assumed to be competent to interpret for a deaf woman, important information may be translated incorrectly. Communication is essential to all maternity care, and even though it may be difficult, it should never be neglected.

Deaf parents have often been deprived of basic knowledge that hearing people take for granted. During their schooling, they may not have learnt about pregnancy and childbirth. They do not have access to radio, not all television programmes are subtitled and often their literary skills are limited because of delayed educational development. With this in mind, midwives have a duty to inform and teach deaf people about the maternity services. School programmes of childcare and sex education exist in which midwives are involved, but these are rarely used in deaf schools or clubs. Unless deaf people are informed about the available maternity services and the choices of care and carer, they will continue to present for maternity care ill informed and ill prepared.

The case history featured below gives an indication of the possible problems faced by a woman with hearing impairment and the steps taken by midwifery staff to meet her needs.

Case history

Mary was 20 years old and had been deaf since contracting meningitis in early childhood. Her hearing was profoundly affected, and her speech was barely audible and quite difficult to understand. She had learned to lip-read. She had previously booked for maternity care in another area, and transferred to the Manchester area when already 26 weeks pregnant.

Mary was married – her husband could hear – and they had developed their own sign language as well as relying on lip-reading. She had a very supportive (hearing) mother, who often accompanied her to the antenatal clinic. It was considered important to arrange for the installation of a baby alarm in Mary's home prior to the birth, and here we encountered a problem. She and her husband were looking for a flat, and in the meantime were living in a rented caravan. Without a permanent address, the baby alarm could not be installed, but a portable model designed for hospital use was borrowed for her. Staff arranged for Mary to take this with her when she went home with the baby and use it on a temporary basis. Fortunately, the couple were able to move into a flat 6 weeks before the baby was born. The social services department organised a system of flashing lights for the doorbell and at the same time installed the baby alarm in readiness for mother and baby's homecoming.

Mary's knowledge of pregnancy and birth was sketchy, and she preferred not to attend group classes. Arrangements were made for her to be taught on an individual basis when she attended for antenatal care. The physiology of birth was explained using diagrams, and this was linked to how Mary would feel, the options for positions in labour and the available methods of pain relief. Teaching was slow, with plenty of time for repetition, to ensure that Mary had at each stage fully understood what was being explained to her.

Antenatal preparation

Antenatal teaching on aspects of pregnancy, childbirth and parenting must be adapted to accommodate the communication needs of couples where one or both partners are deaf. Large classes may be difficult for them if background noise interferes with their hearing aids, class interaction is missed or the teacher's face is not clearly visible. If deafness developed before speech was learnt (prelingual deafness), speech may be poor or difficult to understand, and the deaf person may feel inhibited among others.

Video material is beneficial provided it has sign language interpretation and subtitles. Manufacturers of antenatal teaching material too often disregard the very real needs of deaf people, feeling that meeting them is not economically viable. If a sufficient number of midwives were to demand sign language and subtitling before purchasing or using video films, suppliers might change their priorities. Subtitled material, whether or not it contains sign language, should be no less useful for the hearing viewer, and midwives might do well to bear this in mind and bring it to the notice of manufacturers.

Written material, leaflets and books may be useful to some deaf people, providing they have adequate reading skills. However, these should never be used as a substitute for good personal antenatal teaching, which will probably be best on a one-to-one basis. Any practical teaching will take longer, and time must be allowed for this. To avoid confusion, the midwife should remember to talk to the parents and then demonstrate without talking. This is important because if the teacher talks while demonstrating, the deaf person does not know whether to watch the teacher's face or look at what is being shown.

Continuity of care by a known midwife or a small group of midwives is appreciated by all women and particularly by the woman with hearing impairment. Known midwives will be better able to meet the woman's individual needs and deal with her deafness, her communication needs and her specific worries.

Communication with deaf people is important, but communication is a two-way process, and deaf people should have access to midwives, GPs, health visitors or maternity units by teletext machines ('Minicoms'). These machines are relatively cheap and, when installed in maternity units or health centres, allow deaf people telephone access to health professionals. Some models have printers and can act as answerphones, while others are portable and can be used by community midwives to maintain contact with a deaf client.

Access to maternity units is sometimes hazardous for deaf people. If they are unable to telephone, or the unit does not have a Minicom system, they are unable to announce their arrival. Because of increased security, particularly at night, many maternity units are locked, using intercom or coded access systems. Such intercoms present an additional barrier for the deaf woman trying to gain access when in labour. Midwives should be aware that this is a problem for their deaf client, and arrangements should be made to ensure that contact can be made quickly and easily. A home birth or a domino birth may be suggested as a reasonable option.

Intrapartum care

Care during labour involves adapting maternity care to meet specific needs. Particular attention must be afforded to lighting. Delivery rooms are usually brightly lit to illuminate, for example, the perineal area, but this often casts a shadow on the midwife. Shadows inhibit lip-reading and the transmission of facial expressions, and prevent communication. It is useful to take opportunities to experiment with different positions before labour actually starts. Good lighting and the use of mirrors will increase the flexibility of choice in labour.

Pain relief is very important for all women, perhaps particularly so for those who are deaf as they may have to rely solely on visual methods of communication. The deaf woman in labour should be made aware that some forms of analgesia may cause drowsiness. Drugs such as pethidine should not necessarily be restricted, but the woman must be made aware that they may inhibit her ability to communicate.

The quality of the earlier preparation will make itself clear during labour, as Mary's story indicates.

Case history

Continuity of care for Mary was achieved by her having contact with just three midwives during her pregnancy. All three were involved in her ante-natal care, and one was available when she was admitted in labour. Mary found this helpful. The team of three had ensured that Mary had received relaxation instruction during her pregnancy, and each member had prac-tised this with her. It was particularly good to be able to continue this when her labour began and she and her husband arrived at the hospital.

Mary's labour lasted only 6 hours. She chose to have an epidural sited when her cervix was 4 cm dilated, and she found this form of anaesthesia beneficial, as the pain had begun to make her very tense. She had specifi-cally chosen not to receive pethidine for pain relief, in view of the possible drowsiness that this could cause.

Mary laboured well, and was keen to be fully involved and co-operative. Her eyes watched the midwife continuously, and she commented after-wards that the antenatal teaching had been tremendously helpful. Not only had her known midwives been able to explain fully the processes of labour and what would happen, but one of them was also there with her when these processes unfolded and the teaching was confirmed.

Mary's baby boy was born normally and suckled at the breast almost immediately. His birth weight was 3.2 kg (7 lb).

Postnatal care

Once the baby is born, it is essential that deaf parents gain their indepen-dence by learning how to care for the baby. Advice on feeding, bathing and other routine care should cover the same ground as for hearing mothers, but additional strategies, such as properly used, fluent sign language (Bowles 1991; Lewis 1991) or additional time being taken to demonstrate techniques, may be needed.

Independent care of the baby includes knowing when it is crying. Baby alarms are available (through social services departments) which have a

small microphone placed in the baby's cot to activate flashing lights elsewhere in the home. Portable models can be used in the hospital to help
mothers gain confidence. It should be remembered that there may be a
delay before these alarms can be supplied and installed in the home, and
an application to the appropriate authorities should therefore be made
early in the antenatal period.

Case history

Mary experienced no problems in the postnatal period. During the pregnancy, her known midwives had discussed her preferences about where
she should be nursed after the birth – in a side room, or in the main ward
with the other mothers. This discussion is important, as deaf people are
very light sensitive and Mary could have found that the bed-lights of the
other mothers prevented her from sleeping. In the event, she chose to be in
a side room, where she could practise using the baby alarm.

It is often tempting, when caring for a deaf mother and her newborn
baby, to tell her when her baby is crying. This does nothing to promote her
own independence. Mary had her portable baby alarm in her side room.
She soon learned to respond to its light and would ring the call bell to show
that she had responded. The staff were particularly concerned that Mary
should not feel isolated, and she said she found this support when the baby
alarm went off reassuring. She went home on the fourth day, with her
confidence in her ability to care for her new baby increasing.

The key members of the midwifery team would have liked to continue
visiting Mary once she was discharged from their care but she lived too far
from the hospital. Her mother kindly telephoned, however, with the information that Mary was managing very well and, through her social worker,
had contacted another deaf mother for mutual support and friendship.

This is an important aspect of postnatal support. It is well documented
that new mothers with normal hearing often feel isolated at home with a
new baby (Holden 1990), and for deaf parents it can be considerably
worse. They may be completely unaware of the signs of postnatal depression, and because they think that admitting to feeling depressed will be a
reflection on their ability as a parent, they are often too frightened to ask
for help. Adequate prior knowledge of the possibility of postnatal depression can alleviate this.

SUMMARY

The midwife is uniquely placed to inform, support and be 'with women'
who are themselves hearing impaired or whose baby is expected to be so. In

order for the 'Changing Childbirth' report's (Department of Health 1993) recommendation for woman-centred care to be fully implemented, midwives must take up the challenge of responding to the special needs of these mothers with well-informed strategies.

Midwives can go some considerable way towards helping hearing parents to come to terms with deafness in their infant and showing them how much they can help their child's development and adjustment. The midwife's role lies not only in the provision of information and support, but also in ensuring good communication across the multidisciplinary team and suggesting referrals to specialist professionals where appropriate.

Reviewing the care provided for Mary may show how, with a little thought, midwives are able to provide even a profoundly deaf woman with sufficient information to enable her to make the right choices about her maternity care, promoting self-reliance, confidence and independence. Hearing loss may be a disability in the hearing world, but midwives should no longer see it as a barrier to 'able' parenting.

REFERENCES

Bowles BC 1991 Breastfeeding consultation in sign language. *Journal of Human Lactation* **7**(1):21

Department of Health 1993 *Changing Childbirth. A Report of the Expert Maternity Group.* London: HMSO

Hodnett ED 1994 Support from caregivers during childbirth. In Enkin MW, Keirse MJNC, Renfrew MJ, Nielson JP (eds) *Pregnancy and Childbirth Module, Cochrane Database of Systematic Reviews:* Review No. 03871. Oxford: Cochrane Updates

Holden JM 1990 Emotional problems following childbirth. In Alexander J, Levy V, Roch S (eds) *Postnatal Care.* Basingstoke: Macmillan

Jackson L 1990 The happiest time of your life? *Soundbarrier* **43**:10–11

Kelsall J 1993 The practicalities of improving maternity care for deaf people. In *Proceedings of the International Confederation of Midwives 23rd International Congress,* May 1993, Vancouver, **2**:991–9

Kelsall J, King D, O'Grady D 1992 *Maternity Care for the Deaf.* Edinburgh: Scottish Workshop Publications, Donaldsons College

Kirkham MJ 1986 A feminist perspective in midwifery. In Webb C (ed.) *Feminist Practice in Women's Health Care.* Chichester: John Wiley

Lewis V 1991 *A Good Sign Goes a Long Way.* London: Royal National Institute for Deaf People

McNiven P, Hodnett E 1992 Supporting women in labour: a work sampling study of the activities of labour and delivery nurses. *Birth* **19**(1):3–8

Nolan M 1994 Care for the deaf mother. *Modern Midwife* **4**(7):15–16

Robertson NRC 1986 *Textbook of Neonatology.* Edinburgh: Churchill Livingstone

FURTHER READING

East Berkshire MSCC Consumer Sub-group/NCT ParentAbility 1994 Services and Support for Deaf Parents. An information pack for midwives at Heatherwood and Wrexham Park Hospitals

Kelsall J 1992 She can lip-read, she'll be alright. Improving maternity care for the deaf and hearing-impaired. *Midwifery* **8**(4):176–83

Kelsall J 1993 Giving midwifery care for the deaf in the 1990s. *Midwives Chronicle* **106**(1262):80–2

Lewis V (1990) *Some Experiences of Deaf Mothers.* London: Royal National Institute for Deaf People

USEFUL ADDRESSES

National Childbirth Trust: ParentAbility
Alexandra House
Oldham Terrace
Acton
London W3 6NH   Tel: 0181–992 8637

Royal National Institute for Deaf People
135 High Street
Acton
London W3 6LY   Tel: 0181–993 4748 (voice);
                         0181–993 4691 (Minicom).

Teletec International
Sunningdale House
49 Caldecotte Lake Drive
Caldecotte Business Park
Milton Keynes MK7 8LF   Tel: (01908) 270003
                         For information on teletext communication
                         links (Minicom).

CHAPTER SEVEN

Sexual violence and midwifery practice

Jenny Kitzinger

This chapter examines the ways in which childhood sexual abuse can influence women's reactions to pregnancy, childbirth and the transition to motherhood. Drawing on in-depth interviews with adult survivors, the chapter explores the links between women's experiences of sexual violence and their experiences of giving birth. It describes how such adult life events can stir up strong feelings about past abuse, and it draws out the implications of this for midwifery practice. Finally, the chapter suggests ways in which midwives can help pregnancy and childbirth to be an empowering rather than a disempowering process, which challenges rather than reinforces the feelings of violation and pollution inflicted on women by sexual violence.

THE RESEARCH FINDINGS

The research reported here involved in-depth, tape-recorded interviews with 40 women who were survivors of (mainly incestuous) childhood assault. My interest in the impact of sexual violence on women's lives grew out of my voluntary work in a refuge for young women who had to leave home to escape abuse. It was also fuelled by some research I was then doing into the maternity services (Green *et al.* 1988), as well as by conversations about this issue with my mother, Sheila Kitzinger (see S. Kitzinger 1992).

The research was designed to explore the process of surviving childhood sexual abuse (J. Kitzinger 1990) and it soon emerged that women's experiences of health care could be particularly problematic.

Encounters with health carers in general (from dentists to surgeons), and encounters with the maternity services in particular, were often the source of renewed trauma. In fact, over half of the interviewees reported that such experiences had in some way reminded them of their abuse.

The impact of sexual violence on women's feelings about their bodies is now well documented in the literature written by, and for, survivors (Maltz & Homan 1986; Armstrong 1987; Bass & Davis 1988; Hall & Lloyd 1989).

The following discussion focuses on sexual assault during childhood; however, some of the issues are also relevant for women raped in adulthood.

The consequences of abuse can include hatred for and dissociation from one's own body and can affect a woman's feelings about her reproductive capacity. If women detest their own bodies or feel alienated from their sexual organs, the intimate intrusions of a physical examination can make them feel particularly vulnerable. Their past abuse may also have made them acutely alert to any situation in which they are vulnerable and therefore open to victimisation. The women I interviewed (unless otherwise indicated, all quotations are taken from these interviews) frequently described their reluctance to surrender to intimate manipulations of their bodies while in the powerless position of a patient. Sophie, who was abused by her grandfather, explained, 'I have enormous resistance to opening my legs on demand'.

Although some survivors do not find examinations difficult, others can cope only by 'switching off': 'Of course I hate them, but I just detach my mind from my body, I've had years of practice doing that – with my stepfather!' Some women find that vaginal examinations bring memories of abuse flooding back. One woman, for example, had a flashback after being examined, in which she felt herself to be a child again and re-experienced an assault. Another is fearful that male staff might take advantage of her vulnerability in order to abuse her, so she prefers always to be treated by women. A third talked of her unexpected terror before a vaginal examination when she became convinced that the doctor was going to thrust his whole hand inside her.

For some women, these fears mean that they avoid attending for internal examinations, cervical screening or antenatal care. Morag, now in her forties, managed to avoid vaginal examinations during 16 years on the oral contraceptive pill and throughout a pregnancy. Her evasion of medical care, originally a reaction to her childhood sexual abuse, was reinforced by the treatment she received when, at 20 years old, she had a cervical smear. In a letter written to me after her interview she described her feelings:

> I can see myself walking out of the hospital gate feeling guilty, not a good wife, dirty, in pain, humiliated. They were holding me down while the doctor tried to take a smear; they were shouting at me. It was painful. I just wanted to get away. They said my marriage wouldn't last and I should be ashamed of myself for carrying on like that. When I started to struggle they should not have held me down. It does not seem a big thing but the feelings are still there.

Such behaviour by staff is clearly abusive, but sociologists have pointed out that hospital institutions can encourage such treatment. Staff are sometimes 'paternalistic' and medical institutions routinely 'infantilise' patients (Cartwright 1976; Roberts 1985). Sometimes women feel their own needs are disregarded, that they are treated as 'walking incubators' (Oakley 1986). Ironically, some of the rituals designed to desexualise encounters with health carers (such as a lack of eye contact or the isolated focus on a woman's genitals) can actually make women feel depersonalised and treated 'just like an object'. When women are treated in this way while being subjected to painful and intrusive examinations, this replicates experiences of childhood abuse.

Labour and delivery and the accompanying medical treatment can be frightening, and a woman may feel trapped just as she did when she was pinned down by her assailant. As one woman explained, her labour recalled her abuse because 'I was on my back where I don't like to be, and I was out of control, and I was in pain.' In fact, many women (whether or not they have been sexually abused) talk about unpleasant experiences of birth using the language of rape – they talk of feeling 'skewered', 'abused', and 'treated like a lump of meat' (S. Kitzinger, 1992). For women who have been sexually assaulted in the past, childbirth may feel, as one commented, 'like being sexually abused all over again'. One woman vividly described how her birth experience echoed her childhood victimisation: 'The same indignities, lack of control, humiliation, and depersonalisations. My despair led to a total loss of self-esteem and I attempted suicide... My horror of hospitals and doctors has increased. I find myself terrified at the thought of an examination.'

Midwives may find that they have to deal with the 'fall-out' from women's past experiences or their encounters with doctors. Some incest survivors may approach childbirth as if they are totally helpless; they may be utterly subservient and unable to express their own desires. Others regard the midwife as a potential assailant. They refuse to negotiate and insist on rigid rules about what the midwife can or cannot do. They react to any deviation from pre-agreed plans as if it is an immense betrayal of trust. This can leave midwives feeling that their own professionalism, and indeed character, is being called into question.

It is important to recognise the ways in which a woman's willingness to trust anyone (and perhaps especially health carers) may have been altered by the abuse. Survivors have, after all, been tricked and abused by those, such as a father, who claimed to have their best interests at heart, and they sometimes also feel betrayed by their mothers because they believe that she must have known what was happening. A survivor knows how trust can be abused. She has no reason to have faith in anyone until they have demonstrated just how trustworthy they can be; she is unlikely to accept promises at their face value or to trust a midwife simply because she is a professional. After all, abusers include respected members of the community (including teachers, lawyers, psychiatrists and health professionals), who sometimes use quasi-medical justification for the abuse they inflict on their victims. Miranda's father would insist on putting his fingers in her vagina 'to check you are still a virgin', Diane's father would pull her knickers off 'to make sure you are growing properly' and Lesley's 20-year-old brother raped her when she was 11 under the guise of 'playing doctor'.

Understanding the ways in which trust has been undermined allows the midwife to work with the woman on those issues and to respect her point of view. As Simkin (1992, p 225) points out, 'What is sometimes exasperating and unreasonable to the caregivers really makes all the sense in the world when we recognise why she may have trouble giving up control... The first step for caregivers is to be aware that recollections of sexual abuse can come up unexpectedly and unconsciously during pregnancy and childbirth and can exert powerful effects on the woman. With this awareness comes a different perception of the "difficult" or "demanding" or resistant or over-anxious woman. We realise that she has very good reason to feel the way she does'.

Labour and delivery may have particularly significance for survivors because of the physical sensations involved. A woman may feel as if 'the memory of the violations during my childhood was locked in my birthing muscles' (Rose 1992) or she may fear 'tearing wide open' during the delivery. Some practitioners suggest that such deep-seated fears can stop labour before it goes beyond a woman's control or may make her opt for elective caesarean section (Simkin 1992). Rose (1992, p 216) describes how, during her delivery, 'my mind was full of images of the rape... I was screaming that it felt like the abuser's penis in me, and begging them to get it out! Thankfully, knowing about my past, they made a strong effort to help me through the experience. Through the haze I heard them saying to me, "You are safe now. You are not being raped. It is not a penis going into you, it is your beautiful baby trying to come out".'

Pregnancy and childbirth also invoke feelings about one's sexuality and one's body – how it looks and feels and whether it is 'good' enough (S. Kitzinger 1985; O'Driscoll 1994). These reactions are complicated by abuse. Women often feel that they have been 'ruined' and that their bodies betrayed them by attracting their assailant or sexually responding to his touch (Maltz & Homan 1986; Wisechild 1988). They cannot believe that their polluted and abused flesh can bring forth a perfect baby. Some girls grow up with the continual anxiety that they might become pregnant; indeed, some do become pregnant by their abuser. Such experiences may colour their feelings during this pregnancy (and each midwife must remember that a woman in her care could be carrying the child of a rapist, including, in some cases, her own father) (Zdanuk *et al.* 1987; Schreuders-Bais 1990; Satin *et al.* 1992).

Many incest survivors also believe that their genitals have been damaged beyond repair, or 'turned inside out' by the years of abuse. The fear of long-term physical damage is, for a minority of women, well founded (Cleveland 1986). However, most children experience a symbolic rather than actual physical distortion. They feel that they must have been physically altered by the abuse because of the sheer pain they suffered as children, and this concern is often fed by an adult tendency to warn children that their bodies are infinitely impressionable and that physical signs will yield up secrets of any 'solitary vice'.

Children are told that if they masturbate, they will get hairy hands, picking their nose will make it swell up to twice its natural size, and if they suck their thumb, they will get buck teeth. Young women in the incest survivors' refuge often asked questions such as 'When I get married, will my husband be able to tell?' or confided worries about being 'abnormal', 'all red and swollen' or 'with bits hanging out'. Many women grow up with no access to information about what 'normal' genitalia look like. This, combined with a reluctance to examine that shameful part of themselves (their private parts are 'untouchable' at least by them) means they have little recourse but to live with this fear for years.

It is not only lack of information or the physical experiences of penetration that may influence a survivor's relationship to her body; her feelings are also influenced by the abuser's attitude toward her. He may have called her names ('slut', 'tart', 'whore'); he may have treated her as both dirty and irresistible. The child thus experiences her growing body as it is reflected through the eyes of her assailant. His furtive approach to rubbing her genitals or the way he spits on his fingers before inserting them into her can increase feelings of self-disgust. Any sexual response to his touch can make her despise herself, and if he seems irresistibly attracted by her pubescent body, she may have grown to loath her developing breasts and genitalia. Alison, for example, describes her feelings:

> I can remember cutting my labia with scissors. I can remember shaving my pubic hair... I always wanted to change my genitals. Even though I used to go through my mom's nursing books and knew this was the way they were supposed to be, somehow they never looked right... I know where the feelings stem from. They stem from [the offender] who started his business as soon as he discovered I had pubic hair. Things were never the same after that... He would frequently make the comment 'now you're growing into a woman' as though I was supposed to share his fascination with the idea. (quoted in Jehu 1988, pp 270–1)

These negative images of their genitals obviously have implications for women's feelings about antenatal care and labour, especially for specific procedures such as vaginal examinations, episiotomies and perineal suturing. Pregnancy and labour can thus reawaken anxieties: 'What will the midwife discover when she examines me?'; 'Are there any scars?'; 'Is my vagina wide enough to let the baby come out?' However, by the same token, this can be an opportunity for women to gain information about their bodies and begin to see their sexual organs in a new light. Some women I interviewed spoke of their relief to discover that they were not 'deformed', and, for many, talking with a midwife had been their first opportunity to ask questions about 'down there'. The midwife may be able to offer reassurance that there has been no physical damage or, if there are signs of the abuse, discuss this openly. Women who are scarred should not be treated to averted eyes, and evasion when they seek information. Midwives need to think carefully about how to describe any damage to the genitals. Evasion or negative language can reinforce women's alienation or sense of 'freakishness'. One woman, for example, was informed that she was 'deformed' rather than that she had a ring of scar tissue – perhaps in an effort to deny sexual abuse and the types of injury that might ensue (Courtois & Riley 1992).

In addition to all the issues related to pregnancy and childbirth, a woman may find that feelings about her abuse are stirred up by the fact that she is now the mother of a baby girl or boy. The transition to motherhood confronts women with questions about what it means to be a parent. It is often a time when women think about their own childhood, and it may arouse their fears about the dangers facing their own children. One interviewee's first thoughts after giving birth to her daughter were: 'Oh my God! It's a girl. I can't bear it if she has to go through what I've been through'. Another found that she could not trust her husband with the baby. As she explained: 'My mum didn't know my dad would abuse me when she married him – how do I know my husband won't turn out like that?'

Some women also worry that they themselves are a threat to children. Survivors are repeatedly bombarded with messages that their sexuality is dangerous. The media often refer to incest survivors as 'time-bombs' who are trapped in 'the cycle of abuse', destined to repeat their victimisation by assaulting their children. Such myths fail to address even the simplest flaw in that equation – that most victims of sexual abuse are female and most abusers are male. Given the ubiquitous nature of such theories, however, it is not surprising that survivors are sometimes wary of touching their babies. The sensuality of breastfeeding may provoke anxiety, and daily care incites fears because, as one woman commented, 'They tell you that if you've been abused, you abuse'. Referring to the difficulties she had in bathing her son, she added, 'I didn't like to touch his bits because I thought if I did I'd end up like my dad and do it to him.'

On the other hand, a woman may find holding her own baby brings home the vulnerability and 'innocence' of the infant and makes her feel that she was less to blame for her own childhood abuse. For others, this does not happen until their child reaches the same age as they were when the abuse began. As one mother of a 7-year-old boy commented, 'If he wanted a cuddle you don't take it as he wants sex. I think it's helped having Tim to see what a seven year old looked like'.

Some women also found that becoming a mother made them decide to 'sort themselves out'. As Amy explained, 'I'd think "so what? You are feeling pain – it doesn't matter – you are depressed, so what?" Before I had any children I could live quite happily with the fact. "So, that happened, it doesn't matter, it's a secret." But when I had children... I knew I had to do something about it.'

Given all the factors discussed above, it is not surprising that women often start to talk and seek help during this time (Haugaard & Repucci 1988), and several autobiographical accounts address the links between abuse and postnatal depression (McNeill 1986; 'Fay' 1989). But childbirth *can* be an opportunity for women to relate to their bodies in new ways, to experience them as powerful, competent, and creative.

Although vaginal examinations can reawaken anxieties, they can also be a source of information. Treatment from staff can make women feel powerless and humiliated, but it can make them feel respected and in control. Becoming a mother can make women feel frightened and incompetent, but it can also make them more aware of their own 'childhood innocence' and look toward the future with optimism. Many interviewees spoke positively of the care with which midwives, doctors and nurses responded to their needs. A gentle examination, a listening ear and a respectful approach can all help women to 'reclaim' their bodies and to become angry instead of ashamed of what has been done to them in the past. Sensitivity on the part of staff who understand and validate their distress, provide information, and offer practical support is vital in helping women through such experiences. The following guidelines suggest some ways in which midwives can begin to address this issue.

GUIDELINES FOR MIDWIVES

1. It is essential that all health care staff are informed about sexual violence. This involves reading about the subject and trying to ensure that the topic is discussed in education programmes and in the maternity unit (see Further Reading at the end of the chapter).

2. It is important that midwives be open to the possibility that any women they are caring for may have been sexually assaulted. Some writers recommend routinely asking questions about sexual abuse of all 'patients' (Courtois & Riley 1992). I believe that this is intrusive and may provoke unnecessary anxiety. In any case, some women prefer not to think about their abuse. However, it may be appropriate to introduce the topic in antenatal discussions and to ensure that leaflets about abuse are available. Ignoring the issue only reinforces women's feelings of isolation and freakishness. Contact the local Rape Crisis Information Centre or Citizens Advice Bureau for advice about

leaflets, support groups and helplines to which women can be referred
(Westcott 1991).

3. Respect a woman's desire for confidentiality. Discuss with her whether
there is anyone else (such as her partner or members of the medical
team) with whom she would like to talk about the issue.

4. Be aware of women's fears about 'telling'. Survivors may be reluctant
to talk about their victimisation because of the stigma surrounding it
or because they fear the consequences of revealing such a terrible
secret (their abuser may have threatened them to ensure their silence,
they may have been rejected by other people in whom they have
confided or they may simply not wish to confront their past).

5. Do not force women to explore this subject. Midwives can show a
willingness to discuss sexual violence, but it must be the woman who
decides whether she wishes to take advantage of this. Just because
pregnancy and childbirth are a time when women may have
heightened awareness about their own abuse, this does not mean that
this is necessarily the best time to explore the issue. (Breitenbucher
1991).

6. Accept the woman's pain and distress. Do not try to minimise the impact
of the abuse on her. Survivors are frequently subjected to hollow
reassurance or told that they should have 'got over it' by now (because it
was a 'long time ago' or because the abuse 'wasn't that bad').

7. Recognise that an act that is defined as medical treatment or 'health
care' can still be a form of abuse. Respect a woman's subjective
experience of such treatment and, if necessary, be prepared to help
her to challenge abusive behaviour from other staff. It seems that some
health care providers act as if abuse 'explains away' women's
resistance to examinations or treatment. One midwife overheard a
colleague challenge a 'difficult' woman by asking, 'What's the matter
with you then? Have you been abused or something?' Experience of
abuse does not mean that women's concerns are 'illegitimate' or
distorted, nor should the accusation of having been abused be used
against women in this way.

8. Remember that it is not up to midwives to unearth and diagnose
abuse. Women may have strong reactions to their treatment *whether
or not* they have been sexually abused in the past.

9. Some survivors of childhood sexual abuse seem to become classed as
'difficult patients' by their health care workers. It is important that
midwives and doctors deal with their own feelings of impatience or
frustration and respect any woman's resistance to trusting them. It is
vital to be open about the power dynamics that exist (within the
maternity services, for example) and not to make false promises.
Anything which the woman experiences as a betrayal of trust may
only reinforce her feelings of being abused.

10. Think about your own reactions. Midwives sometimes find that they are left with feelings of distress, anger, or grief, or memories of their own experiences of sexual violence. It is also very disturbing for the midwife when a woman experiences flashbacks during labour or examinations. You may find it helpful to talk through your feelings with a colleague.

11. Survivors of child sexual abuse may be fearful for their babies' safety. Women who were abused themselves are often particularly aware of the dangers to young children. Do not dismiss these fears. Point out that this can be positive if it makes them more likely to take precautions and provide information to their children. Discuss plans of action that might help to protect the woman's children. Such plans may involve anything from introducing children to the range of books about abuse at an appropriate age to being sure that the baby is not left alone with the man who abused the mother – such as the baby's grandfather.

12. Survivors of child sexual abuse may need extra support to establish breastfeeding, and it is important to acknowledge the 'normality' of sensual responses to the baby.

13. Consider the language used during antenatal classes or during labour. For example, some women find that relaxation sessions or 'listening' to their body may lower their defences, exposing them to horrific memories of abuse. As Simkin (1992, p 225) points out, 'Using language and imagery emphasising "tuning in," "yielding", or "surrendering" to the contractions, or "listening to your body" may distress the woman whose body has been a source of anguish'. If a woman is very aware of the effects of abuse, ask her about the strategies she usually employs to cope with frightening recollections or how she deals with 'flashbacks' and 'dissociation'. During labour, it may be important to encourage her to 'stay in' her body, to maintain eye contact and to remind her that she is safe.

Think through each aspect of your practice from the point of view of a woman who has been sexually assaulted. For example, consider all the issues involved in a vaginal examination. Acknowledge that many women find the examination difficult. Explain how, why and for how long you will examine her. Knowing why the examination is being done, and what it involves, directly contrasts with the incomprehension and confusion she experienced as a child. Explicitly state that you will stop the moment she asks, and discuss her preferred position for the examination. Make sure she has the opportunity to talk about what she found helpful or unhelpful about the way you examined her and to ask any questions, for example about her own genitalia. (Some women find it useful to see photographs demonstrating the variety of women's genitalia.) Above all, listen to the woman: she is the best source of information about what she would prefer, and it is impossible to generalise about the best way of responding to every woman.

14. Finally, all the recommendations suggested above are influenced by the conditions of midwifery education and practice. Discussion of sexual violence should be built into midwifery education programmes, and midwives need the working conditions and institutional support that enable them to learn about the issue and spend time with individual women. Above all, midwives need the power to act as advocates for the women in their care and the freedom to provide the continuity of care that will enable them to build up trust and understanding.

SUMMARY

Instead of seeing survivors of sexual abuse as women with 'special needs' who can be identified and offered 'special treatment', it is perhaps better to consider sexual violence as a continuum that influences all women's experiences of their bodies.

In North America, random population surveys show that between 12 and 38 per cent of adult women have experienced some form of childhood sexual abuse, while British researchers report rates between 16 and 42 per cent (Kelly 1988; Kelly *et al.* 1991). One study of 535 young women who had become pregnant during adolescence found that 44 per cent had been raped (Boyer & Fine 1992).

The variation between the statistics reflects variable factors, such as the definitions of 'child' and 'abuse' and the sensitivity of the research design, but the research evidence suggests that sexual violence in one form or another is widespread, and many of us know how it feels to be sexually harassed, intimidated, pressurised into sex or physically humiliated at some time in our lives. The threat or reality of rape affects us all. The women quoted in this chapter had endured childhood experiences that had long-term effects on their sense of self, and the quotations reflect the voices of those who had the strongest reactions to the events surrounding pregnancy and childbirth. Many of the interviewees experienced less dramatic reactions and most did not discuss the issue with their health carers. Thus it is important to realise that survivors of abuse cannot be identified as a discrete group.

Instead of thinking of survivors as posing 'special problems', it then becomes more appropriate to think about the insights that they can bring to the maternity services. Each of the factors that are so often important to survivors of sexual violence – communication, information, respect, choice and control – are important to all women.

Survivors' reactions throw a spotlight on the impact of sexual violence on women's relationship with their bodies and highlight the power dynamics of the encounter between women and health care professionals. Their insights help us to explore the construction of childbirth within a world in which women are routinely subjected to a variety of abuses and within which the hospital institution and medical hierarchy can further disempower both 'patient' and midwife. The challenge is to ensure that midwifery care helps to counteract rather than re-enact the violation of women's bodies.

REFERENCES

Armstrong L 1987 *Kiss Daddy Goodnight*. New York: Pocket Books

Bass E, Davis L 1988 *The Courage to Heal: A guide for women survivors of child sexual abuse*. New York: Harper & Row

Boyer D, Fine D 1992 Sexual abuse as a factor in adolescent pregnancy and child maltreatment. *Family Planning Perspectives* **24**(1):4–11, 19

Breitenbucher J 1991 Commentary: Sexual abuse issues should not be addressed in childbirth education classes. *International Journal of Childbirth Education* **6**(4):33

Cartwright A 1976 *Patients and Their Doctors*. London: Routledge & Kegan Paul

Cleveland A 1986 *Incest: The story of three women*. Lexington, MA: Lexington Books

Courtois C, Riley C 1992 Pregnancy and childbirth as triggers for abuse memories: implications for care. *Birth* **19**(4):222–4

'Fay' 1989 *Listen to Me: Talking survival*. Manchester: Gatehouse Projects

Green J, Coupland V, Kitzinger J 1988 *Great Expectations: A prospective study of women's expectations and experiences of childbirth*. Child Care and Development Group: Cambridge University.

Hall L, Lloyd S 1989 *Surviving Sexual Abuse*. London: Falmer

Haugaard J, Repucci N 1988 *The Sexual Abuse of Children: A comprehensive guide to current knowledge and intervention strategies*. San Francisco: Jossey-Bass

Jehu D, in association with Gazan M, Klassen C 1988 *Beyond Sexual Abuse: Therapy with Women who were Childhood Victims*. New York: John Wiley

Kelly L 1988 *Surviving Sexual Violence*. Cambridge: Polity Press

Kelly L, Regan L, Burton S 1991 An Exploratory Study of the Prevalence of Sexual Abuse in a Sample of 16–21 Year Olds. Child Abuse Studies Unit, Polytechnic of North London

Kitzinger J 1990 Who are you kidding? Children, power and the struggle against sexual abuse. In James A, Prout A (eds) *Constructing and Reconstructing Childhood*. London: Falmer Press

Kitzinger S 1985 *Woman's Experience of Sex*. Harmondsworth: Penguin

Kitzinger S 1992 Birth and violence against women. In Roberts H (ed.) *Women's Health Matters*. London: Routledge & Kegan Paul

McNeill P 1986 And some of us went mad. In McNeill P, McShea M, Parmar P (eds) *Through the Break*. London: Sheba Press

Maltz W, Homan B 1986 *Incest and Sexuality*. Lexington MA: Lexington Books

Oakley A 1986 *The Captured Womb*. Oxford: Blackwell

O'Driscoll M 1994 Midwives, childbirth and sexuality. *British Journal of Midwifery* **2**(1):39–41

Roberts H 1985 *The Patient Patients: Women and their doctors*. London: Pandora

Rose A 1992 Effects of childhood sexual abuse on childbirth: one woman's story. *Birth* **19**(4):214–18

Satin A, Ramin S, Paicurich J 1992 The prevalence of sexual assault: a survey of 2404 puerperal women. *American Journal of Obstetrics and Gynecology* **167**(1):973–5

Schreuders-Bais C 1990 The Incest Pregnancy. Paper given at the World Congress on Child Abuse and Neglect, Hamburg, September 1990

Simkin P 1992 Overcoming the legacy of childhood sexual abuse: the role of caregivers and childbirth educators. *Birth* **19**(4):224–6

Westcott C 1991 Sexual abuse and childbirth education. *International Journal of Childbirth Education* **6**(4):32

Wisechild L 1988 *Obsidian Mirror: An adult healing from incest*. Seattle: Seal Press

Zdanuk J, Harris C, Wisian N 1987 Adolescent pregnancy and incest: the nurse's role as counsellor. *Journal of Obstetrics, Gynaecology and Neonatal Nursing* March/April: 99–104

FURTHER READING

Bass E, Davis L 1988 *The Courage to Heal: A guide for women survivors of child sexual abuse*. New York: Harper & Row

Courtois C, Riley C 1992 Pregnancy and childbirth as triggers for abuse memories: implications for care. *Birth* **19**(4):222–4

Kitzinger J 1990 The internal examination. *The Practitioner* **234**:698–702

Kitzinger J 1990 Recalling the pain: incest survivors' experience of obstetrics and gynaecology. *Nursing Times* **86**(3):38–40

Kitzinger S 1992 Birth and violence against women. In Roberts H (ed.) *Women's Health Matters*. London: Routledge & Kegan Paul

Rose A 1992 Effects of childhood sexual abuse on childbirth: one woman's story. *Birth* **19**(4):214–18

Simkin P 1992 Overcoming the legacy of childhood sexual abuse: the role of caregivers and childbirth educators. *Birth* **19**(4):224–6

CHAPTER EIGHT

Young mothers

Pippa MacKeith and Rosemary Phillipson

Is being a young mother any different from being any other mother? 'Teenage mothers' often find themselves on the receiving end of adverse publicity – 'irresponsible', 'dependent on the State', 'jumping the queue for council housing', 'unmarried and therefore immoral' – yet the majority are successful as parents, often in difficult circumstances.

This chapter will look at why some young people embark on parenthood earlier than others, and at the effect that adolescence has on their role as parents. It will explore the ways in which socioeconomic factors influence the lives of these young families and why the majority are living in poverty. Finally, the chapter will consider the sort of midwifery service that can best serve the needs of this group of young parents.

IDENTIFYING THE CLIENT GROUP

The terms 'teenage pregnancy' and 'teenage mother' are in common use in headlines, in the media and in professional discussions. The image these phrases conjure up is of a schoolgirl, a single mother, and a mother and child at risk. It is necessary to look more closely at the messages that these labels convey about this group. Who are these 'teenage mums'?

Conception rates and birth rates for different ages within the teenage years vary dramatically. The total number of conceptions and births in the under-16s represents a very small proportion of all teenage conceptions; the majority of teenage conceptions occur at the ages of 18 and 19 years (Figure 8.1, Table 8.1). However, it must be acknowledged that, although the conception rate for girls under 16 is very low, it is significant and has shown a gradual increase throughout the 1980s. In 1991, this rate went down for the first time in 10 years, but remained higher than the rate for 1981 (Tables 8.2 and 8.3).

To put teenage conceptions into perspective, it is necessary to recognise that the number of conceptions in the under-20 age group is one of the lowest of all the age groups (Tables 8.2 and 8.3), and that only a proportion lead to births (Table 8.4 and Figure 8.2).

Figure 8.1   *Conception rates per 1000 women aged 14–19 years, 1981 to 1991 (data from OPCS Conception Series FM1 No. 21)*

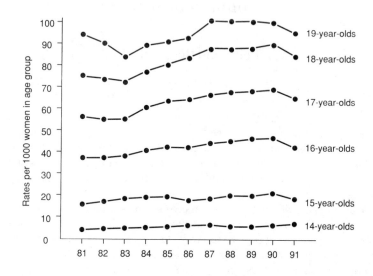

Table 8.1   *Conception rates per 1000 women aged 14–19 years, 1981 to 1991 (data from OPCS Conception Series FM1 No. 21)*

			Age (years)			
Year	14	15	16	17	18	19
1981	4.6	15.8	37.7	56.8	76.2	94.0
1982	4.9	17.1	37.6	55.8	74.0	90.1
1983	5.4	18.3	38.7	55.9	72.1	84.9
1984	5.5	19.1	41.8	61.2	77.6	89.2
1985	5.6	19.2	42.4	64.0	80.4	91.4
1986	5.7	18.6	42.1	64.8	83.3	93.2
1987	5.8	19.7	44.4	67.4	87.7	100.6
1988	5.7	20.4	45.2	68.1	87.4	100.0
1989	5.9	20.7	46.0	68.8	87.2	100.4
1990	6.5	21.5	46.3	69.4	89.2	100.5
1991	6.6	19.8	43.4	65.3	84.6	95.6

Table 8.2   *Conception rates per 1000 women in different age groups, 1981 and 1991 (data from OPCS Conception Series FM1 No. 21)*

Age (years)	1981	1991
Under-16s *	7.3	9.3
Under-20s †	57.1	65.1
20–24	128.9	120.6
25–29	132.7	135.0
30–34	68.4	89.4
35–39	25.9	34.0
40 and over ‡	7.2	6.4

*   Rates per 1000 women aged 13–15 years.
†   Rates per 1000 women aged 15–19 years.
‡   Rates per 1000 women aged 40–44 years.

Table 8.3   *Conception rates per 1000 women by age group, 1981 to 1991 (data from OPCS Conception Series FM1 No. 21)*

			Age (years)				
Year	Under 16s*	Under 20s†	20–24	25–29	30–34	35–39	40 and over‡
1981	7.3	57.1	128.9	132.7	68.4	25.9	7.2
1982	7.8	56.4	127.1	134.1	69.7	25.8	6.9
1983	8.3	55.9	122.2	133.6	71.4	26.0	6.7
1984	8.7	59.8	124.4	137.9	75.6	26.7	6.6
1985	8.7	61.7	121.6	135.9	77.4	26.5	6.4
1986	8.7	62.3	122.2	137.2	80.2	27.2	6.3
1987	9.3	66.2	126.4	138.6	82.6	28.9	6.4
1988	9.4	66.9	125.0	136.1	83.7	30.0	6.4
1989	9.4	67.8	124.6	137.8	87.3	31.8	6.4
1990	10.1	69.1	124.4	137.8	89.1	33.2	6.4
1991	9.3	65.1	120.6	135.0	89.4	34.0	6.4

*   Rates per 1000 women aged 13–15 years.
†   Rates per 1000 women aged 15–19 years.
‡   Rates per 1000 women aged 40–44 years.

Society sends confused messages about the 'right' time to have a baby, putting women in a 'no-win' situation. Society condemns women for having children while they are young, but obstetricians suggest that the optimum physical age for childbirth is 18–25 years (Towler & Butler-Manuel 1980; Morris 1981). Those women who delay motherhood and have a career risk disapproval when they wish to continue with their career and return to their paid work instead of staying at home with their children. They also experience difficulties in securing appropriate, affordable childcare to meet their needs (Phoenix 1991). It is only those in well-paid jobs who can have the 'luxury' of using the limited childcare facilities available.

The time at which women choose to have a baby is influenced by many complex factors. Class and culture can influence whether or not a teenager goes on to become a young mother, an issue discussed in the section on Active Choice of Motherhood, below.

Table 8.4   *Number of conceptions leading to maternities by age group, 1991 (data from OPCS Conception Series FM1 No. 21)*

Age	No. of conceptions (000s)
All ages	688.4
Under-16s *	3.8
Under-20s †	67.8
20–24	182.4
25–29	243.5
30–34	143.5
35–39	44.4
40 and over ‡	6.9

*   Rates per 1000 women aged 13–15 years.
†   Rates per 1000 women aged 15–19 years.
‡   Rates per 1000 women aged 40–44 years.

Figure 8.2   *Total number of births (in thousands) for England and Wales 1991, showing the under-20s and the under-16s as a proportion of the total (data from OPCS Conception Series FM No.21)*

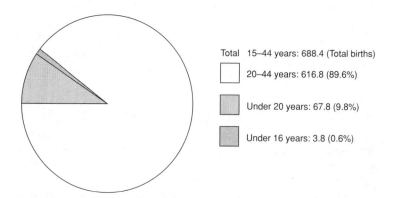

Total   15–44 years: 688.4 (Total births)

20–44 years: 616.8 (89.6%)

Under 20 years: 67.8 (9.8%)

Under 16 years: 3.8 (0.6%)

SEX

There are many factors that may influence a young person's decision to have sexual intercourse for the first time. Contrary to popular belief, offering sex education at an early age does not encourage sexual intercourse (Barth *et al.* 1992). In the Netherlands, where sex education is widespread, not only do the young people start sexual activity no earlier than their British contemporaries, but in addition there is a much lower rate of teenage conception (Jones *et al.* 1985). As well as comprehensive sex education, the Netherlands has an accessible family planning service that gives high priority to maintaining confidentiality. There is a general acceptance of teenage sexuality.

In England and Wales, the majority of 16–24-year-olds have had their first experience of sexual intercourse at the age of 17 years; however, 20 per cent of 16–19-year-olds report that they have had sexual intercourse before their 16th birthday (Johnson *et al.* 1994). Society needs to accept that sexual activity in young people is inevitable (Jones *et al.* 1985). In order to achieve a low conception rate, an acceptable and accessible family planning service should be made available (Hudson & Ineichen 1991).

Factors that influence sexual behaviour include the media, families and peer pressure. In the media, minimal messages are given about the consequences of sex. Portrayal of sex and sexuality is ambiguous, shown on the one hand as unrealistic and romantic and, on the other, as violent (RCOG 1991). Families can have positive or negative influences, with a wide range of attitudes towards sexuality and sexual behaviour.

There may be a willingness to talk about sex-related issues, but this can be hindered by not having appropriate shared language and vocabulary to communicate between generations. Some families are unwilling to discuss these issues and rely on other agencies, such as schools, to address all areas relating to sex and sexuality. Other families may see any discussion on these issues as being inappropriate.

Young people are more susceptible to peer group pressure, and this may include pressure to become sexually active earlier than they would otherwise have chosen. Some young women feel themselves to be less powerful than their male partners (Phoenix 1991), and this may affect their decisions about when to start having sexual intercourse, whether to use contraception and what method of contraception to use (Holland *et al.* 1990).

CONTRACEPTION

It is important to remember that young people do not fit neatly into one single mould. They are not a homogeneous group. It may be necessary to provide a range of services to meet the needs of this diverse age group.

Decision making about contraception may be influenced by factors similar to those involved in deciding when to begin sexual activity (for example, media influences, familial attitudes, peer group or partner pressure). In order to meet the Health of the Nation target of reducing pregnancies in the under-16-year-olds, it is essential to provide contraceptive services that are seen as appropriate and acceptable, enabling young people to make informed choices.

Jones *et al.* (1985) found confidentiality to be a most important issue in every country. In the UK, nearly 75 per cent of under-16-year-olds and 50 per cent of 16–19-year-olds were worried that the doctor would tell their parents (Allen 1991). In 1991, of all 15-year-olds estimated to have had intercourse, less than one quarter had visited a family planning clinic (Allen 1991). It is unlikely that many of the remaining three-quarters consulted their own GP for their contraceptive needs, as all the indications are that young teenagers are reluctant to do so (Holland *et al.* 1990).

Several factors to be taken into account when planning contraceptive services for this age group are:

• confidentiality – as mentioned above, this is vital;
• the provision of a drop-in facility, as priorities fluctuate – this enables young people to use the service opportunistically without a lot of planning;
• the attitude of the staff, which should be accepting and non-judgemental;
• anonymity – provision of a service away from the client's own neighbourhood, family and friends, for example in the centre of a town or city;
• session times – these should be suitable to most of the client group rather than at the convenience of the professional group;
• communication skills – staff should be good listeners and be able to use young people's own language, thus enhancing communication.

ACTIVE CHOICE – MOTHERHOOD

It is important to recognise that a significant number of young women in their teenage years make an active choice to become mothers (Family Planning Service 1991). Provision of good sex education and accessible contraceptive services is unlikely to affect these young people. The choice of whether or not to become a mother is a complex one, and the influences are multifactorial. This, of course, can be said for women of all ages and not just for those in their teenage years (Oakley 1979; Dowricks & Grundgergs 1980; Sherr 1995). It must be remembered that the majority of teenagers who choose to have a baby are 18 or 19 years old.

The use of the blanket term 'teenage mother' might be assumed to imply that early motherhood is uniformly distributed throughout the teenage years. This is in fact not the case... In England and Wales in 1980, 18 and 19 year olds accounted for nearly two thirds of mothers under 20 years of age, and those under 17 years of age accounted for less than a fifth. (Phoenix 1991, p 54)

Culture within differing social class influences expectations of young women. Young mothers are more likely to come from families in which their own mothers had given birth to their first child under the age of 20 years. With friends and relatives also having children while young, they live in an environment where young motherhood is seen as the norm (Phoenix 1991).

Pregnant young women who go on to have their babies and those who have abortions are different in many ways. Of those who continued with their pregnancy, the majority were opposed to abortion as an option. Women choosing an abortion tended to be of higher social class, with better academic achievements and more ambition. The Thomas Coran Research Unit study showed that most women in further education had not wanted to become pregnant when they did (Phoenix 1991). It would appear that this group of women have a vision of their future that does not necessarily involve motherhood.

Many young women who go on to become young mothers have been shown to have experienced difficulties in obtaining employment. Their prospects are poor, and as they intend to have a baby at some time in the future, they see no valid reason for deferring motherhood.

An incorrect view, too often supported by people in powerful positions, is that young women get pregnant in order to get a council house or in order to claim welfare benefits (*Guardian* 1993; Chartered Institute of Housing 1993). The Thomas Coran Research Unit, in its study of teenage women, found that no one had such an ulterior motive. This was duplicated by a study in which women expressed derision and disbelief at such an idea (Clarke 1989).

Wilson and Neckerman (1987) found that births to young women living in poverty did not increase and decline in line with changes in welfare policy. They therefore concluded that women do not become pregnant in order to obtain welfare benefit.

POVERTY AND HEALTH

Young mothers get a bad press. Teenage pregnancy is invariably identified as a problem and is seen not only as a moral problem, but also as a health problem. According to Mills (1990), teenage mothers are at higher risk of anaemia and of having low birthweight babies, but complications in labour are no higher than for more mature mothers. Konje *et al.* (1992) report little difference between the health of pregnant younger teenagers and that of pregnant women in their early twenties, although they found that there was an increased incidence in the younger age group of anaemia, urinary tract infection and hypertension.

In socioeconomic terms, teenage pregnancy is associated with high levels of disadvantage for both mother and child. However, studies in Britain and America are revealing that poor outcomes are by no means inevitable. Many teenage mothers and their children achieve good levels of educational and occupational progress (McIntyre & Cunningham-Burley 1993). Although children of teenage parents are at higher risk than others of illness and accidents, several studies have found that age itself is not a significant factor (Butler *et al.* 1981; Makison 1985; Carlson *et al.* 1986).

Many young mothers live in poor housing. Some are homeless or in temporary accommodation (Simms & Smith 1986; Blackburn 1991), others in grossly unsuitable accommodation. They live on very low incomes, many relying on state benefits. The report 'Poor Expectations' produced by NCH, Action for Children and the Maternity Alliance found that benefit levels were insufficient to sustain a pregnant women on a healthy diet (Dallison & Lobstein 1995).

Poor housing and low income are known to affect health outcomes (SCOPH 1994). When young mothers and their children are compared with families living in comparable circumstances of poverty and deprivation, it becomes clear that it is not age but socioeconomic circumstance that is the major factor resulting in less than favourable outcomes.

Having a child at an early age is not itself a cause of poverty (McIntyre & Cunningham-Burley 1993). Most young mothers will already have left school without obtaining any educational qualifications. They will also have had difficulties finding a job. The fathers of their babies may have had similar experiences and often cannot contribute financially. Opportunities for further education or stable employment are limited for both young men and women.

Once they have had a child, some young women become motivated to improve their employment prospects and to seek further education. Ironically, they then encounter barriers such as insufficient and inappropriate facilities for childcare and limited access to suitable opportunities (Phoenix 1991).

The links between poverty and health must be understood. Midwives need to acknowledge that parents often have the information but not the means to improve the health of their family. A study by Mayall (1986) into child health care showed that all mothers were similar in their perception of what promoted good health. They all accepted personal responsibility for their child's health but found that their material circumstances prevented them from achieving the high standards they would wish for their children.

Blackburn (1991) makes it clear that families on low incomes have as much knowledge about health issues (for example, about what constitutes a healthy diet) as do other people in the UK. As one young woman put it:

> The baby could have had better nourishment before he was born if I'd had enough money to be able to eat properly, and now I'm breast feeding he would get better fed if I was [better fed]. (Salfield 1985, in Blackburn 1991)

The majority of women who smoke are aware of the health risks of smoking. They are also women living on low incomes. Health education antismoking campaigns have been targeted at low-income groups but have had little effect on smoking behaviour. Evidence suggests that women smoke in order to help them cope with the stress of living in poverty (Graham 1992; see also Chapter 4 in this volume). Smoking can help them economise, for example, by suppressing the feelings of hunger. One lone mother has summed up thus:

> I think smoking stops me getting so irritable. I can cope with things better. If I was economising, I'd cut down on cigarettes but I wouldn't give up. I'd stop eating... Food just isn't that important to me but having a cigarette is the only thing I do just for myself. (Graham 1987, in Blackburn 1991)

It is important to remember that the difficulties young mothers experience are due more to the material circumstances in which they live than to their age.

TRANSITION TO ADULTHOOD

Pregnancy brings about rapid bodily changes that women of all ages can find difficult to accept. In addition to this, young pregnant women are still coming to terms with the physical changes that have been brought about through puberty. The impact on an individual will vary depending upon the physical or psychological stage of development at which she gets pregnant. Both pregnancy and puberty can result in women feeling that they are no longer in control of their own bodies.

For many young women in this age group, great importance is given to being able to assert their identity through body image and fashion, which gives them membership of their chosen peer groups. A young pregnant woman is eventually unable to wear the 'right' clothes and fully participate in the activities in which her friends are involved. This can have a drastic effect on her self-esteem and can result in feelings of isolation.

In our society, the transition from childhood and adulthood is ill-defined. In some cultures, there are rites of passage for this time, such as celebrations around the onset of menstruation (Gabriel 1974). In our society, it can be confusing at times when we treat young people as children one minute and shortly afterwards expect a much more mature 'adult' attitude. This confusing pattern continues for young mothers, with family and professionals telling them what to do and expecting them to respond accordingly – then expecting them to be independent and autonomous, and to know what to do with their children. These mixed messages can contribute towards undermining a new mother's self-confidence.

MIDWIVES

Midwives and young mothers generally share the same aims – the outcome of a healthy mother and a healthy baby. However, their means to achieve this may differ. It is important for midwives to acknowledge these differences and to look at ways of working together with young mothers to achieve positive outcomes. Young as she is, the woman should feel that she has control over her own care. According to the document 'Changing Childbirth', she should be:

> the focus of maternity care. She should be able to feel that she is in control of what is happening to her and able to make decisions about her care, based on her needs, having discussed matters fully with the professionals involved. (Department of Health 1993)

At a given time, the midwife's priority might be to carry out an antenatal check to assess the wellbeing of a pregnant young woman. On the other hand, the woman's priority might be to visit the DSS office to ensure that she receives this week's benefit payment. For the young woman and her growing baby, this decision to sort out her finances is a positive health choice as she needs food and warmth to survive. Midwives should acknowledge that there are basic primary human needs (provision of warmth, food and shelter) that must be met before a woman can address other issues (Maslow 1970).

Midwives not only want a healthy mother and baby, but also a mother who has sufficient confidence in herself and her ability to care for a new baby. A confident mother is more likely to be able to make the appropriate choices regarding her own and her baby's health and to use the health service effectively. Midwives can play an important role in helping to increase a woman's self-confidence and self-esteem.

Midwives must be careful that, as well-meaning professionals, they do not inadvertently undermine a young woman's confidence: it can be too easy to offer help that may disempower the woman, leaving her feeling that she is no longer in control. The young woman herself may assume that the midwife, along with the rest of society, disapproves of her and her pregnancy. This is why, from the first contact, the midwife's attitude to teenage women is so important.

Midwives who are judgemental achieve nothing positive. Instead they reduce self-esteem, inspire resentment and destroy the relationship with the client. Generally, young women want to trust their midwife and the maternity services. To achieve this, one of the first steps is to recognise the importance of the role young women are playing – in caring for themselves in pregnancy, and in the 24-hour care of a new baby. They should be offered the positive reinforcement and encouragement that all mothers need.

Midwives must be careful to avoid giving generalised praise, which can become insincere when overused. They need to look more closely at each individual woman and give her credit for her own specific areas of competence. It is *always* possible to find something that a mother is doing well.

Relationships can take time to develop between a young woman and a midwife. The midwife needs to listen to what it is that her client wants from her. It may be difficult for the woman to express how she feels. There may be many barriers; she may feel that she is disapproved of. She may lack confidence, although this might be masked by a precocious façade. She may have had previous negative experiences of the health service. She is new to adulthood and might find it difficult to admit to being scared, as this makes her feel like a child again. She may believe that 'adults aren't scared, adults can cope'.

It is important for midwives to be patient and to use their counselling skills. They need to listen well and help women to work out their own priorities and solutions or simply allow them to 'offload'. This is not always possible in a busy clinic where there is much pressure and little time. Midwives need to think about how they can best get to know clients in a situation free from pressure and frustrations, where they can feel safe and relaxed.

In order to do this, we need to look at our own practice, the facilities and resources available to us and how we make best use of them. For example, would it be better to use a local community centre for a clinic rather than a hospital or health centre? For one woman, a home visit might provide an ideal setting, but for another it might be totally inappropriate owing to lack of privacy. It is important to ensure that maternity services are easily accessible to all groups (Department of Health 1993). Perhaps we could consider inviting teenage clients to attend at either the beginning or end of a clinic, and building in extra time for them. We need to be flexible in our approach.

We could provide a more informal setting at clinics, where refreshments are available and discussion encouraged. It may be that a 'drop in' session at which we make ourselves freely available could be the most appropriate service in a given area. This might initially seem an ineffective use of time. What if no one were to turn up? But if the midwife arranges to have other work at hand, such as completing records or preparation for antenatal groups, she will be able to feel more relaxed and less frustrated when uptake is erratic.

It may be appropriate to have a specific clinic for young mothers and/or a group where the young women could share their expectations and fears and meet other people in a similar situation. Much might be gained from providing an opportunity for antenatal and postnatal young women to meet as they will be able to relate to each other and share experiences (MacKeith *et al.* 1991).

Another way in which young women might raise their self-esteem and feel more in control could be to involve them as much as possible in their own care. For example, they could be taught how to test their own urine, take each other's blood pressure and listen to each other's babies' heartbeats. This can help to demystify antenatal care and stimulate useful discussion.

In labour too, it is important to remember to involve young women in their care. As it is for many older women, it might be easier for a young woman to submit passively to what happens. Her expectations may not appear to be great, but she will have hopes and fears of her own. Labour plans can be useful but may need to be updated as the pregnancy develops and expectations change. Discovering what those fears and hopes are, sharing information fully and encouraging her to decide what would be best for her are the challenges. Where major or minor intervention is needed, a young woman can still be involved in the making of decisions about her care. Having some feeling of control and an understanding of what is happening can help her to come to terms with her experiences at a later date.

How can midwives nurture a young mother's confidence in herself and her new role, that of caring for her child? There must be a balance – all new mothers need to be nurtured, as illustrated by the role of the 'doula' (Raphael 1973, Odent 1992). With a young woman, particularly a very young one, it can be all too easy for a midwife to be overwhelming, to be overprotective, to take over, to make all her decisions for her.

Are we too prescriptive in the way things are done, for example in the way in which we demonstrate bathing a baby? Do we do too much for the mother or make decisions for her? She may have cared for small babies many times before, she might already have a wealth of experience, and if so we need to acknowledge her skills and build on them. How do we assess each mother's needs for support, encouragement and information? Once she is home, how do we ensure that she has appropriate support or adequate living conditions?

Midwives can be flexible in the way in which they offer their service. We cannot change people's lives, but we can ask ourselves whether there are any ways in which we can help. What benefits is this mother entitled to? Could she qualify for better housing? Where can she meet other young mothers? Midwives can introduce women to each other and therefore help to reduce the isolation that can be a major health hazard (MacKeith *et al.* 1991). Midwives should be a great source of knowledge about other agencies available, but need to have a clear understanding of what each service can offer and ensure that referrals are appropriate and effective.

SUPPORT FOR MIDWIVES

Working with young mothers can be quite demanding as they may have special needs apart from those common to all mothers. In any situation where we decide to change our way of practice, there is a challenge, but this can also be frustrating and sometimes frightening. To help us to develop our practice, we all need encouragement and support. Before embarking on changes, it can be helpful actively to seek out support. This might come from a variety of sources. We need to find people who have an understanding of what we are trying to do, as well as others who may have experience in working within this field. We may find the support we need from managers and midwifery colleagues, but it may be necessary to go further afield, for example to youth workers, teachers or community workers. Appropriate support is extremely important (MacKeith *et al.* 1991).

EVALUATION

Evaluating our work is essential. It enables us to learn continually and to modify and improve our practice. Evaluation also provides information about the service we are giving and how effective it is in achieving our goals. Managers need this information in order to give us support for what we are doing. In order to evaluate, we need to be very clear about what we hope to achieve. As discussed earlier, our aims include not only healthy mothers and babies, but also other goals, such as mothers who feel confident in their new role. Quantitive evaluation, for example figures on birthweight and mortality, is relatively straightforward compared with qualitative evaluation in which we measure the less tangible outcomes. Raising self-esteem and alleviating isolation, for example, are difficult to measure, but they are important achievements and can have lasting effects on the long-term health of the family. As midwives, it is important that we ensure that these achievements are given a high profile. Therefore we need to find the means to measure these outcomes so that we can convey their importance to managers and planners.

SUMMARY

The majority of teenage mothers are 18–19-year-olds and are from families with a tradition of early parenthood. Where young women's prospects are poor in terms of employment, they see little reason for deferring motherhood.

Evidence suggests that good sex education and a comprehensive family planning service are effective in reducing the teenage pregnancy rate. Contrary to popular belief, they have no effect on the average age at which young people become sexually active (Barth *et al.* 1992).

Research suggests that poverty rather than age is the main factor affecting poorer outcomes for young families (Butler *et al.* 1981; Makison 1985; Carlson *et al.* 1986).

Adolescence is a time of ambiguity, being an adult and a child at the same time. Being a mother causes further confusion for society, which on the one hand is shocked at the 'child' having a child, yet on the other is expecting adult and responsible behaviour.

Different ways of providing a midwifery service that meets the needs of young mothers include, for example, the importance of attitude and approach, as well as the provision of specialised clinics and groups. There are many ways in which midwives can involve mothers in their own care, and these can lead to a positive working partnership with young people.

Midwives themselves need to be supported, both in this type of work and when changing their practice. It is important to devise appropriate methods of evaluating our service in order to plan and improve services for young mothers. The majority of young mothers work very hard under difficult circumstances and become good mothers. As midwives, we can have considerable influence on this.

REFERENCES

Allen I 1991 *Family Planning and Pregnancy Counselling Projects for Young People*. London: Policy Studies Institute

Barth RP *et al.* 1992 Preventing adolescent pregnancy with social and cognitive skills. *Journal of Adolescent Research* **2**:208–32

Blackburn C 1991 *Poverty and Health – Working with Families*. Milton Keynes: Open University Press

Butler M, Ineichen B, Taylor B, Wadsworth J 1981 *Teenage Mothering*. Report of Department of Health and Social Security. Bristol: Univeristy of Bristol

Carlson DB, Labarba RC, Sclafani JD, Bowes CA 1986 Cognitive and motor development in infants of adolescent mothers: a longitudinal analysis. *International Journal of Behavioural Development*

Chartered Institute of Housing 1993 *One Parent Families – Are they jumping the queue?* Coventry: Chartered Institute of Housing

Clarke E 1989 *Young Single Mothers Today*. A Qualitive Study of Housing and Support Needs. London: National Council of One Parent Families

Dallison J, Lobstein T 1995 *Poor Expectations: Poverty and undernourishment in pregnancy*. London: NCH, Action for Children and the Maternity Alliance

Department of Health 1993 *Changing Childbirth*. A Report of the Expert Maternity Group. London: HMSO

Dowricks S, Grundgergs S 1980 *Why Children?* London: Virago

Family Planning Service 1991 *Summary of information from Form KT31 DH Statistics and Management Information (SM12B).* London: FPS

Gabriel J 1974 *Children Growing Up.* London: University of London Press

Graham H 1987 Women's Poverty and Caring. In Glendinning C, Millar J (eds) *Women in Poverty in Britain.* Brighton: Wheatsheaf

Graham H 1992 *Smoking among Working Class Mothers.* Final Report, Department of Applied Social Studies, University of Warwick

Guardian 1993 Michael Howard (Home Secretary) and Sir George Young (Housing Minister) reported at the Conservative Party Conference. 6/10/93 and 8/10/93

Holland J, Ramazanoglu C, Scott S, Sharpe S 1990 *Sex, Risk and Danger: AIDS education policy and young women's sexuality.* Women's Risk Aids Project Paper 1. London: Tufnell Press

Hudson F, Ineichen B 1991 *Taking it Lying Down: Sexuality and motherhood.* Basingstoke: Macmillan

Johnson AM, Wadsworth J, Wellings K, Field J 1994 *Sexual Attitudes and Lifestyles.* Oxford: Blackwell Scientific

Jones EF, Forrest JD, Goldman N *et al.* 1985 Teenage pregnancy in developed countries: determinates and policy implications. *Family Planning Perspectives* **17**(2)53–63

Konje JC *et al.* 1992 Early teenage pregnancies in Hull. *British Journal of Obstetrics and Gynaecology* **99**:969–73

McIntyre S, Cunningham-Burley S 1993. In Rhode DL, Lawson A (eds) *The Politics of Pregnancy: Adolescent sexuality and public policy.* Yale: Yale University Press

MacKeith P, Phillipson R, Rowe A 1991 *45 Cope Street – Young Mothers Learning through Group Work: An evaluation report.* Nottingham: Nottingham Community Health

Makison C 1985 The health consequences of teenage fertility. Family Planning perspectives **17**:132; cited in Scholl T *et al.* 1987 Pre-natal care adequacy and the outcome of adolescent pregnancy: effects of weight gain, preterm delivery and birth weights. *Journal of Obstetrics and Gynaecology* **69**:312–16

Maslow AH 1970 *Motivation and Personality,* 2nd edn. New York: Harper & Row

Mayall B 1986 *Keeping Children Healthy and Happy.* London: Allen & Unwin

Mills MJG 1990 Teenage mothers. In Alexander J, Levy V, Roch S (eds) *Midwifery Practice: Postnatal care – a research-based approach.* Basingstoke: Macmillan

Morris N 1981 The biological advantages and socal disadvantages of teenage pregnancy. *American Journal of Public Health* **71**(8):796

Oakley A 1979 *From Here to Maternity: Becoming a mother.* Harmondsworth: Penguin

Odent M 1992 *The Nature of Birth and Breastfeeding.* Westport CT: Bergin & Garvey

Phoenix A 1991 *Young Mothers?* Cambridge: Polity Press

Raphael D 1973 *The Tender Gift: Breastfeeding*. Englewood Cliffs NJ: Prentice Hall

Royal College of Obstetricians and Gynaecologists (RCOG) 1991 Factors influencing Reproductive Behaviour, ch 5 in Report of the RCOG Working Party on Unplanned Pregnancy

SCOPH 1994 *Housing, Homelessness and Health*. Standing Conference on Public Health Working Group Report. London: SCOPH

Sherr 1995 *Psychology of Pregnancy and Childbirth*. Oxford: Blackwell Scientific

Simms M, Smith C 1986 *Teenage Mothers and their Partners*. London: HMSO

Towler J, Butler-Manuel R 1980 *Modern Obstetrics for Student Midwives*. London: Lloyd Luke

Townsend P, Davidson N 1982 *Inequalities in Health. The Black Report*. Harmondsworth: Penguin

Wilson W, Neckerman K 1987 Poverty and Family Structure: The widening gap between evidence and public policy issues. In Wilson WJ *The Truly Disadvantaged – the inner city, the underclass and public policy*. London: University of Chicago Press

CHAPTER NINE

Pregnancy following assisted conception

Mary Sidebotham

When a previously infertile couple realise their dream and a pregnancy is achieved, there is very little information available to them, or to the professionals caring for them, on how to cope with the mixed and varying emotions they may experience during the pregnancy. How will they adapt to parenthood? Will the transition from being infertile individuals to parents be difficult or smooth? How may they shed the identity of failure and learn to live with success?

The motivation to reproduce may be instinctive, reflecting a biological need to pass on one's genes (Winston 1987). The survival of the species depends on reproduction. With the introduction of reliable contraception and safe, legal abortion over the past 35 years, women have been granted a degree of control over the process. However, conception is not always as easy as it is expected to be.

There is great social and cultural pressure upon couples to conform and produce a child (Kozolanka 1989). Many individuals may see reproduction as a means of achieving adulthood and may desire a child to give them the chances in life that they never had themselves (Raphael-Leff 1991). Or they may regard the birth of a child as confirmation of their body's normal functioning ability and successful gender role fulfilment (Lasker & Borg 1989). Furthermore, according to Oakley (1986), children are seen as 'the inalienable property of women, symbolising achievement in a world where underachievement is the rule'.

Infertility affects about 1 in 6 of the population. The desire to bear children can be overwhelming, and the distress and grief experienced by couples who fail to conceive naturally can be devastating (Kon 1993). However, there is a wealth of information available for couples who wish to pursue their dream and have a child. Possible avenues for the couple to pursue are given below. When the couple are still at the stage of considering their options, they will find plenty of available information on the possible avenues, including:

- adoption (Toynbee 1985);
- surrogacy (Cotton & Winn 1985; Reid 1988);

- the use of donor gametes in a reproductive cycle (Snowden 1984);
- the *in vitro* fertilisation process itself (Lasker & Borg 1989; Klein 1989).

Because of the relative newness of this field of science, however, there has been very little work published on the subject of parenting *after* infertility, especially following the use of the modern reproductive technology that is currently available. While being based in practical experience, this chapter considers what relevant research there is. Midwives need to have an insight into the emotional pain felt by couples who face a diagnosis of subfertility and the effect that the treatment has upon the couple and their relationship. Midwives must also be aware that these experiences may have a profound effect on the couple's acceptance of the pregnancy and their eventual relationship with their child. The challenge is to know how best to help the couple when problems, either real or potential, are identified. A major part of the midwife's role involves sharing her knowledge and experience of the transition to motherhood. By working in partnership with the couple, she may be able to explain that the same worries and emotions are felt by many other new parents-to be.

INFERTILITY AND EMOTIONS

> Every month my future child bleeds to death, hope is driven painfully away from me because I don't want to let go, I want to hold on. Every month a little miscarriage, an abortion of my hopes. (Belk-Schmehle 1989)

This quotation vividly describes the pain of failed conception. Each month the arrival of the menses can signal a crushing sense of failure in the couple trying to conceive (Mahlstedt 1985). This can have a devastating effect upon their whole lives, altering relationships and personal perceptions, overshadowing everything else. The effect upon one or both partners can be so strong it may even lead to suicide (CIBA Foundation 1986).

When subfertility is diagnosed, the couple often go through a grieving process. All the reactions of shock, denial, anger, guilt, depression and resolution can be found in the literature (Edelmann & Connolly 1986). If investigation identifies one partner as being responsible for the problem, it can cause extreme depression, with a feeling of isolation and failure in that person (Hargreaves Pearson 1992). A loss of body image may be experienced and a sense of failure in the gender role. Men may suffer temporary impotence following diagnosis (Raphael-Leff 1991).

The diagnosis may cause a feeling of resentment and anger in the other partner, be it open or hidden, which may put an extreme strain upon the relationship. The sexual relationship may change as intercourse loses the loving element and becomes a monthly chore. Women are reported as being more likely to exhibit anxieties and negative emotions (Ravel *et al.* 1987). The couple may feel an irrational level of guilt about their infertility, especially if they have had other sexual partners and have suffered from sexually transmitted diseases (Downie 1988). Many relationships are thrown into a state of turmoil and distress.

In the past, choices for such couples were very limited. They had either to resign themselves to remaining childless or to pursue the possibility of adopting a child. Now, with the advances being made in treatment, together with the ever-decreasing number of babies available for adoption, more and more couples are seeking treatment for their infertility (Toynbee 1985; Warnock 1992).

Today, medical science holds out hope, but what appears to be a wide-open avenue of possibilities to conceive narrows as each option fails. The effort becomes funnel shaped, focusing upon the last urgent option, be it *in vitro* fertilisation (IVF) or artificial insemination by donor (AID) (Raphael-Leff 1991). With new treatments, which often have high profile media coverage, becoming available almost annually, many couples believe that their infertility can be cured (Pappert 1989; Hodginkson 1992). They may see the fertility specialist as a last resort, with almost God-like powers to give them a child (Winkler 1989). The treatment programmes can be extremely stressful, even 'dehumanising' (Wood & Westmore 1984). Some couples feel that they have succumbed to social pressures to conform and have thereby been coerced into treatment, leaving no stone unturned in their quest for a child (Jones 1991).

Women feel that their bodies are being manipulated (Corea 1985), and many men dislike the thought of their child being born as a product of masturbation (Lasker & Borg 1989). Some men find it impossible to produce the sperm sample at the required time, further increasing the tensions between the couple (Jones 1991). In some cases, couples in this situation have been asked to make a choice between going ahead using donor sperm or abandoning the treatment programme, without being given the opportunity to discuss this fully (Lasker & Borg 1989).

Not all couples undergoing fertility treatment will conceive the longed-for baby. After IVF, the live birth rate per treatment cycle is around 12.5–13 per cent (12.7 per cent in 1992, according to the Human Fertilisation and Embryology Authority 1994 statistics). As the couples themselves will be aware that only a proportion of attempts at assisted conception are successful, they may have very mixed feelings about other couples on the programme. It is hard to wish the precious successes on others in the same position. No one wants to deny the existence of their own 'phantom baby' who is just waiting in the wings (Raphael-Leff 1991).

Maintaining confidentiality and economic security may also prove difficult for these couples because of the long periods away from work, the potential costs involved and the physical effects of the hormone treatments.

SUCCESSFUL FERTILISATION

After the intensive treatment and attention couples receive from their doctors during the investigation and treatment of infertility, many couples leave the specialist centres once a pregnancy has been confirmed. They then become clients at the local maternity hospital where their full history may not be known. This change may lead to their feeling abandoned as the health professionals with whom they now have contact may have no concept of the magnitude of the fertility problems with which the couple have coped and the stress which will have been caused by the treatment. The couple may feel unable to discuss their doubts and fears with these carers, who see only their success. They have achieved their dream, a viable pregnancy. They may feel (or be made to feel) that they should be grateful, whereas they may in fact be experiencing continued anxiety about the eventual outcome of the pregnancy.

Although these couples will have received professional counselling, as recommended by the Warnock Report (Department of Health 1984), this does not continue once the pregnancy has been confirmed and they have come back into the main system. Even if a need for counselling to continue is identified, the facility may not always be available locally, or it may not be available immediately – an appointment for 6 weeks hence is no help in the immediate present.

The midwife's role

The midwife is ideally placed to help her clients to accept their pregnancy and enjoy it, as well as to provide information and reassurance (Garner 1985; Denton 1996). In order to help the couple who have achieved a pregnancy following infertility treatment, she must be fully aware of the psychological impact of infertility and the emotional, physical and often financial stresses placed upon a relationship by infertility treatment.

Problems identified in the literature to date which are commonly experienced include those associated with what one author describes as 'the tentative pregnancy' (Katz Rothman 1988). The couples concerned have become used to failure, and after what may have been years of trying, they may find it hard to believe that the pregnancy is real and will continue successfully. Dunnington and Glazer (1991) suggest that they may use denial of pregnancy as emotional protection against further potential failure. Garner (1985) suggests that the fear of disappointment, heightened anxiety and denial of pregnancy could cause delayed parent–child attachment, along with a delay in preparing for the child and difficulty in re-integrating parental roles when the child is born.

The denial of pregnancy may delay the development of maternal identity, which Rubin (1984) believes begins during pregnancy. A woman who fails to conceive changes her personal perception. She no longer sees herself as a healthy, fertile female and potential mother. Instead, as each month compounds the feeling of failure, she loses the identity of fertile woman and replaces it with that of infertile woman. Difficulty in believing in the pregnancy may be a defence mechanism against further failure. The woman may be unable to lose her infertile identity, especially as the problem that caused her to develop that identity has been bypassed rather than solved. Once the child is born, she will be infertile again, not a healthy, fertile woman who will become pregnant again normally when she chooses (Dunnington & Glazer 1991).

The midwife who is aware of these potential problems should help the woman to accept and enjoy her pregnancy. It would help if, like any other pregnant woman, she were encouraged to discuss her fears and worries about the pregnancy and her ability to cope when the baby is born. She may find reassurance in being told that most women experience fears and worries at some time during their pregnancies, regardless of the conceptional origin.

It would be helpful if, with the woman's consent, the named midwife or head professional could liaise with the counsellors at the fertility treatment centre. This would enable information about any problems identified before conception to be shared. Together, the counsellor, the woman and her partner could make suggestions to the midwife on how the woman can make the transition from seeing herself as infertile and undergoing treatment, to seeing herself as a healthy woman expecting a baby and being a partner with the named midwife in her own and her baby's care.

The woman's care should be carefully planned by the midwife using one of the theoretical models available (Crichton 1993; Bryar 1995). The spiritual, psychological, physiological and sociocultural needs of the woman and her partner will all need to be taken into account.

These measures should encourage the development of a trusting relationship between the couple and the midwife. The benefits of the therapeutic relationship include early detection of psychological or emotional problems and the opportunity for early advice or referral where necessary.

ANTENATAL SCREENING

Screening for fetal abnormality poses problems that can further affect acceptance of the pregnancy. When there has been a delay in achieving a successful conception, women are more likely to be in the at-risk age group for congenital abnormalities in the fetus. Screening will be offered, and in many cases this will include the Triple test (Decrespigny 1991), a non-invasive procedure that would give the woman a clearer knowledge of her individual risk of carrying a child with Down syndrome. However, should the projected risk of the child being affected prove to be higher than average, the couple will have to make the difficult choice between not accepting any further screening (despite the chance of a higher than average risk of congenital abnormality) or undergoing an invasive procedure such as amniocentesis.

If the couple decline further screening, they will need much support and understanding from their carers during the subsequent months until the child is born and its state of health is known. If the couple do decide to undergo further diagnostic tests, however, it should be remembered that screening itself is based on the assumption that therapeutic termination of pregnancy is an acceptable option. Couples should not be considered for invasive screening unless they have carefully considered the implications of this. The psychological stress of considering terminating a pregnancy that has been so difficult to achieve is enormous. Those who do choose an invasive procedure must also be made aware that in doing so they are accepting a small associated risk of miscarriage in what may be their only successful conception. The couple must be given the opportunity to discuss their worries and should be given honest and up to date information, within the counselling session, on the level of risk involved and the degree of accuracy in testing.

The couple should be supported in whatever decision they make regarding screening, even if it goes against the advice given to them by the professionals. At the appropriate time, the midwife should be in a position to refer the couple to any appropriate support agencies, either to help prepare them for the birth of a handicapped child or to support them following a termination for fetal abnormality.

MULTIPLE PREGNANCY

The incidence of multiple birth is considerably higher after most forms of assisted conception than it is after spontaneous conception. In 1990, there were 20 per cent more twin pregnancies and 4 per cent more triplet pregnancies among couples achieving pregnancy after assisted conception than in the population at large (Kon 1993). This brings with it its own problems (Denton 1996). Parents expecting more than one baby should be given as much information, advice and support as possible (Davies 1995).

In certain circumstances, selective reduction (selective feticide) may be offered to maintain the woman's health and to optimise the chances of the remaining gestation sacs maturing to term (Howie 1990). This procedure should be unnecessary for pregnancies created nowadays as a result of IVF or GIFT (gamete intra-fallopian transfer), as there is now a limit of three or even two eggs or embryos being replaced in any one treatment cycle (Price 1990). However, it may still be a necessary option when the pregnancy is multiple as a result of super-ovulation therapy and may also be considered when one fetus in a multiple pregnancy has a congenital abnormality.

The couple in such a situation will have to make the difficult decision of whether to sacrifice one or more potential children to enhance the chances of survival for the remaining fetus(es). They have to make this choice knowing that the procedure may result in total pregnancy loss. Many individuals suffer long-term depression following selective reduction and will need the non-judgemental support of family, friends and carers at this difficult time to help them cope (Howie 1990).

Provision of fertility treatment on the NHS is not available throughout the UK. Many parents may therefore have already spent large sums of money achieving the longed-for pregnancy. Some may even have sold their house or amassed debts. The realisation that they are not expecting one baby, but two or even three, may therefore increase financial stress at a time when this can be ill afforded. The extra financial burden of a multiple pregnancy may put great strain upon a relationship. Practical help, such as organising a home help when the babies are born, may be necessary. If income support or other benefits are applicable, they should be claimed, and the services of a social worker should be offered where appropriate. The midwife should also refer the couple to the local support agencies (such as the Twins and Multiple Births Association) early in the pregnancy, which can help them to prepare themselves realistically for a multiple birth and offer assistance with the acquisition of baby equipment in cases of need.

The extra medical intervention associated with multiple births is well documented (Ghazi *et al.* 1991; Rufat *et al.* 1994), as is the increased (if sometimes unnecessary) intervention rate with the more mature primagravida (Silverton 1993). Many women pregnant following assisted conception will fall into one if not both of these categories and find themselves exposed to this heightened medical attention. MacFarlane *et al.* (1990) report that the higher obstetric intervention rate can be attributed to the parents' excessive anxieties and the obstetrician's concern with the 'precious pregnancy'. The effects of this on the development of parent–child relationships are also well documented (Bryan 1989; Golombok *et al.* 1995).

NURTURING SELF-CONFIDENCE

Because women often have increased anxiety levels during pregnancy, they may in fact welcome extra attention from the medical team, However, instead of being reassuring, it could have the opposite effect and make the woman worry more. The midwife should recognise this as a potential problem and help the woman to maintain her optimum health during pregnancy by offering advice on diet, exercise and lifestyle. This will increase the woman's sense of wellbeing and thus increase her self-confidence, enabling her to accept her body's ability to nurture the pregnancy and thereby decrease the risk of unnecessary medical intervention.

The midwife must work in close liaison with the obstetrician responsible for the woman's care. Together they should try to achieve a happy medium: a level of intervention to ensure that the mother and fetus receive optimum care, but one which does not provoke unnecessary anxiety. The midwife should also ensure that the woman and her partner are involved in all decision making concerning her care and that they are kept fully informed throughout the pregnancy, labour and puerperium.

When caring for such couples, the midwife should be aware that they may be experiencing conflict with long-held spiritual beliefs, especially if they have decided on treatment against the teaching of their Church (Boyd *et al.* 1986). She must also be aware that some sectors of society and also some members of the nursing and midwifery professions disapprove of the practice and ethics of reproductive technology. The couple may find themselves subjected to this disapproval from family, friends, colleagues and, indirectly, even complete strangers. This disapproval can often be accompanied by painful and personal comment. The midwife caring for couples after assisted conception should consider her own feelings with care and be honest about any prejudices she herself might have. If she is the named midwife caring for a particular woman, her duty is to support the couple concerned with compassion and empathy through what could potentially be a very difficult time for them. If, for whatever reason, she feels unable to this, she should discuss her worries with her supervisor of midwives.

ACHIEVING BALANCED PARENTHOOD

After the birth of a first child, a couple become a family. Raphael-Leff (1991) suggests that couples who wish to make an integrated transition to parenthood need to renegotiate their relationship with each other first. They need to home in on their own nurturing abilities and prepare for child-rearing by analysing their own experience of being parented and resolving any conflicts from the past. This preparation could be difficult for any couple to achieve, but for the couple who have lived through the pyschological trauma of subfertility and its treatment, it may take longer, and they may need more assistance to make the smooth transition to parenthood.

Most of these couples, having reached the point of having a child, report their relationship as being strengthened by the experience, so this should enable them to support each other through the first few difficult months of adapting their lifestyles to care for a new baby.

As discussed earlier, following assisted conception many couples use denial of the pregnancy as an emotional protection against potential failure. If this is not resolved during the pregnancy, the midwife may find herself in the position of having to help them to adapt quickly to the role of parents when the child is eventually born, as it is often only when they take the baby home that many of these couples can accept the reality of their success – that they have a child of their own at last.

LIFE WITH A NEW BABY

Couples who have had difficulty in conceiving a longed-for baby may have particularly high expectations of themselves as parents. Consequently, some may have difficulty in coping with a real child who may not live up to their idealised dream of a perfect baby (Kitzinger 1978). Parenthood may not be as glamorous as expected, and they may be disappointed by their inability to cope with the early parenting experience in general (Raphael-Leff 1991). The midwife must assure them that this is often the case with new parents, and that their confidence and ability to cope will increase each day as the family get used to each other.

Dunnington and Glazer (1991) have shown that previously infertile women expressed a lack of self-confidence in mothering the child, especially with breastfeeding, when compared with never-infertile women. This study also reported role conflict, with previously infertile women experiencing a loss of career identity during the transition to motherhood. These negative feelings could contribute to the higher levels of postnatal depression experienced by women who have had infertility problems (Kumar 1982). However, Bernstein *et al.* (1988) stated that although previously infertile women do have raised levels of depression, hostility and interpersonal sensitivity, indicating mild distress, these do not indicate serious dysfunction. However, they found that men demonstrated lower levels of hostility, possibly reflecting the healing effect of the social recognition of manhood that fatherhood conveys.

During the antenatal period, the midwife will have had the opportunity to help couples prepare realistically for life with a newborn baby. After what may have been years of avoiding being with parents of young children because of the pain it caused them, previously infertile couples will have been encouraged to mix with such people, to experience what they are really like. They should have been encouraged to join antenatal preparation groups, such as those run by the National Childbirth Trust, aquanatal classes, and local parentcraft and relaxation classes. The purpose behind joining these groups is twofold. First, the education and health benefits derived from belonging to such groups are found by many women to be valuable. Second, the groups provide an opportunity to mix with other pregnant women. Friendships often form within these groups, which can provide a valuable support network after the babies are born.

Attendance at postnatal support groups should be encouraged to continue to develop circles of friends and peers started during the antenatal period. Such groups are often initiated by the midwife and continued by the health visitor.

If the woman's career has played an important part in her life prior to giving birth, and she plans to return to work, the midwife and health visitor should give the help and information she needs, including details of local childcare facilities. If she expresses feelings of guilt at leaving her much-loved and wanted baby at home, she should be reminded that most women in the same situation will have the same feelings and that this is an entirely normal reaction. However, she may need support as she comes to terms with these feelings.

ATTITUDES TO DONOR GAMETES

Problems with the transition to parenthood have been identified in couples where donor gametes have been used, suggesting that a missing genetic link between the child and one or both parents may subsequently affect interfamily relationships (Golombok 1992). Provision is made within the Human Fertilisation and Embryology Act 1990 13(6) for the couple who receive treatment services that involve the use of donated eggs, sperm or embryos to be given a suitable opportunity to receive counselling that will be directed towards the implications of taking this proposed step (Morgan & Lee 1991). This should address the couple's ability to accept the child as 'theirs' rather than 'his', when donor eggs are used, and 'theirs' rather than 'hers', when donor sperm is used. Goode and Hahn (1993) feel that the mother's biological attachment through pregnancy offsets her lack of genetic attachment should donor eggs be used. The child in these cases will usually be considered 'theirs'.

Where donor sperm is used, the father's involvement should be encouraged throughout all stages of the pregnancy and childrearing process. This will help him to accept the child as his despite the lack of a genetic link. Section 28-2 of the Human Fertilisation and Embryology Act 1990 gives legal recognition to the child and states that the woman's husband who consents to her treatment with donor sperm will be legally recognised as the father.

Along with having to resolve their own feelings of accepting treatment using donor gametes, the couple will have to decide whether to tell family, friends, and ultimately the child of its conceptional origins. Some couples cannot accept the stigma of people knowing that the child has been born as a result of reproductive technology, and it can be even more difficult for those who have been treated using donor gametes or embryos (O'Donovan 1990). This is especially relevant when the parents feel that such knowledge may affect the child's acceptance into the wider family circle by grandparents, aunts, uncles, etc.

TO TELL OR NOT TO TELL?

Popular opinion seems to support the argument that everyone should have the right to be able to establish details of their identity as an individual human being (Morgan & Lee 1991). The advice given by social workers to parents of children conceived using AID is to share details (O'Donovan 1990). Those children in the future who are told of their conceptional origins will be able to apply to the Human Fertilisation and Embryology Authority for limited, non-identifying information about the gamete donor. This information may include such details as physical characteristics, education, occupation and general family health. The Authority will also disclose whether the child could be genetically related to a prospective partner.

Despite conventional wisdom supporting the right of the child to know its conceptional origins, it is still a very difficult decision for the parents to make. There is very little published research on the effect of conceptional origins on the psychological development of the child(ren) concerned. One can only study the experience of adopted children and those born following AID to help the parents to decide what to tell their children. If they do decide to maintain confidentiality, it may be very difficult to explain the pregnancy to family and friends who knew of the fertility problem, especially if the woman is known to be menopausal or the man to be infertile.

This may be a very stressful time for the new parents. The midwife must work within the UKCC Code of Practice and maintain confidentiality as demanded by the UKCC Code of Professional Conduct, but she could also direct the parents to counselling services, where available, to help them to see the wider aspects of their decision and help them prepare for any possible consequences of that decision. If they decide not to tell the child, they may always worry that he or she may find out accidentally. The consequences of this occurring for children born as a result of egg donation or IVF are largely unknown. This is an area in need of further research (Ethics Committee of the American Fertility Society 1990; Golombok 1992).

POTENTIAL DEVELOPMENT OF THE CHILD

Little is known on whether the intense media attention that surrounds such children or the conceptional origin in itself has any effect upon their physical and psychological development. It is known, however, that children born as a result of reproductive technology may be treated differently by their peers from those conceived normally. Friends may tease them because they 'came out of a test-tube' (Lasker & Borg 1989). Their parents have waited a long time for their 'miracle baby' and invested much of their time, finances and lives into the child's creation. Parental expectations of the child have been shown to be very high; they are often overprotective, worrying excessively about the child's health and development, treating the child as extra special and finding it hard to let go and allow the child to develop a sense of independence (Lasker & Borg 1989; Jones 1991). The associated media hype that still surrounds these births does little to protect the family's right to privacy and may prompt the parents to continue treating the child in this way.

The children may find themselves unable to live up to their parents' high expectations and may display emotional and behavioural problems. Golombok *et al.* (1995) say that it may be that when children conceived by the new reproductive technologies develop psychological problems. the parents may attribute these problems to the conceptional origins. They then treat the child differently from parents who conceived their child naturally, who are able to look at the problem from a wider angle rather than concentrating on the one thing that makes their child different from the rest.

It is not only the parents who will be watching these children very carefully. The researchers in the field of reproductive medicine will also be studying this small select sample of children, as it is not known whether the procedures involved in this new field have a direct effect on the child's development (Medical Research Council 1990; Golombok *et al.* 1995). The small studies published to date, which include those by Mushin *et al.* (1986), Yovich *et al.* (1986) and Golombok *et al.* (1995), show that the children are intellectually developing well. However, they demonstrated a higher rate of emotional and behavioural problems among these children when compared with their peers in a nursery class. The levels of behavioural problems found were similar to those found in social services day nurseries and were more common among boys.

The midwife's role

The midwife can help to make the parents aware of the fact that these children are developing normally. If they maintain the friendships they made during pregnancy, they will be able to see other children of the same age, which will help them to accept that all children develop at their own pace but that milestones will eventually be reached. They will also be able to discuss any problems concerning the child's development and behaviour with other mothers who will probably have conceived naturally, and who are likely to be experiencing the same problems. This helps the couple realise that their child is not really any different from the rest, and they can then be more relaxed in their approach to childrearing, thus reducing the higher levels of emotional and behavioural problems identified by Golombok *et al.* (1995).

The role of other health professionals is crucial, too , as the family move from the care of the midwife into that of the health visitor. The health visitor is likely to be the main port of call for advice about any aspects of the child's development and behaviour that may give the parents cause for concern.

FUTURE DEVELOPMENTS IN THE FIELD

Pressure is increasing, internationally, to remove the secrecy from gametic donation. There is pressure in the USA and elsewhere for more information to be released, and in Sweden this has led to legislation (O'Donovan 1990). If the parents are given more information about the donor, it may help them to accept their child's behaviour and development as normal for that individual child, rather than trying to attribute any inconsistencies to genetic origins.

The number of centres offering treatment for subfertility problems is increasing, and appeals are being made by support groups such as ISSUE and CHILD (see address list below) to increase provision within the NHS (Kon 1993).

As the number of people receiving treatment increases, so also will the number of children being born as a result. All midwives will be expected to care for these women and should be able to base that care on current research findings (Bryan & Higgins 1995).

There does appear to be a consensus of opinion among the experts that the subject of parenting after infertility is in need of further research. Woollett (1989) suggests a need for more information on the transition to parenthood in terms of counselling needs. Dunnington and Glazer (1991) suggest the need for further research to fully understand the impact of infertility on early mothering behaviour.

Midwives should rise to the challenge and use their developing experience gained while caring for these women to pursue topics in this field of science, in research projects of their own. It is only by asking the relevant questions, and doing longitudinal studies with families already created by the new reproductive technologies, that we will be able to reduce the anxieties of the families currently involved and improve the experience for the families of the future.

SUMMARY

The number of pregnancies now resulting from assisted conception techniques is increasing all the time. However, most couples who have achieved a pregnancy by such a method then become consumers of the NHS maternity services like any other prospective parents. They may choose not to identify themselves as previously infertile couples, or they may not be given the opportunity to do so.

The midwife has a key role to play in supporting, advising and preparing the woman and her partner throughout the pregnancy, delivery and early postnatal period. The named midwife is the woman's key link professional and as such should be prepared to act as guide, friend and advocate at a crucial time in the woman's life.

The midwife needs to understand that the couple may have difficulty coming to terms with the reality of the pregnancy and is uniquely placed to help them to redefine their self-concept from that of 'infertile couple' to 'prospective parents'. The midwife should give the woman and her partner space to express their anxieties about the pregnancy itself, and about how they will manage as parents after the baby's birth. This may be particularly necessary if more than one baby is expected.

The parents-to-be will need to be informed about the various organisations that can offer them support, be it practical, educational, social or financial. The midwife should ensure that she has the relevant up to date information available.

Should the parents be in one of the 'target groups' for invasive procedures, such as diagnostic techniques or selective reduction, the midwife will need to be particularly supportive and empathic as she gives the couple the information and the time necessary to make the decision that is best for them.

Once the baby has been born, the mother may be at risk of postnatal depression or she may have difficulty bonding with the real child. The midwife should be alert to the woman's state of mind and emotions and, as the key link professional, may be the first person to notice whether specialist referral is indicated.

The challenge to today's midwife is to allow the woman to be a full partner in her own care. In a situation such as pregnancy following assisted conception, months, perhaps years, of feeling passive and disempowered, of having things 'done to her', might have been experienced before the achievement of a pregnancy. In such situations, the midwife's role in undoing some of these negative experiences and restoring the woman's sense of dignity and 'normality' is crucial.

REFERENCES

Belk-Schmehle A 1989 Every month a little miscarriage. In Klein RD (ed.) *Infertile Women Speak Out about their Experience of Reproductive Medicine.* London: Pandora Press

Bernstein J, Mattox J, Kellner R 1988 Psychological status of previously infertile couples after successful pregnancy. *Journal of Obstetric, Gynaecologic and Neonatal Nursing* Nov/Dec: 404–8

Boyd K, Callaghan B, Shotter E 1986 *Life before Birth. Consensus in Medical Ethics.* London: SPCK

Bryan EM 1989 Ethical dilemmas and multiple births. *Midwife, Health Visitor and Community Nurse* **25**:236–40

Bryan E, Higgins R 1995 *Infertility: New choices, new dilemmas*. Harmondsworth: Penguin

Bryar R 1995 *Theory for Midwifery Practice*. Basingstoke: Macmillan

CIBA Foundation 1986 *Embryo Research, Yes or No*. London: Tavistock

Corea G 1985 *The Mother Machine*. New York: Harper & Row

Cotton K, Winn D 1985 *Baby Cotton for Love and Money*. London: Dorling Kindersley

Crichton MA 1993 Assessment of Needs Model for Midwifery Care. Unpublished MA thesis, Victoria University, Manchester

Davies M 1995 Educating parents for multiple births. *Modern Midwife* **5**(11):10–14

Decrespigny B 1991 *Which Tests for my Unborn Baby? A Guide to Prenatal Diagnosis*. Oxford: Oxford University Press

Denton J 1996 Pregnancy after treatment for infertility. In *Midwifery Practice: Core topics 1*. Alexander J, Levy V, Roch S (eds) Basingstoke: Macmillan

Department of Health 1984 *Report of the Committee of Enquiry into Human Fertilisation and Embryology (The Warnock Report)*. London: HMSO

Downie S 1988 *Baby making – The Technology and the Ethics*. London: Bodley Head

Dunnington R, Glazer G 1991 Maternal identity and early mothering behaviour in previously infertile women. *Journal of Obstetric, Gynaecologic and Neonatal Nursing* **20**(4):309–16

Edelmann RJ, Connolly KJ 1986 Psychological aspects of infertility. *British Journal of Medical Psychology* **59**:209–19

Ethics Committee of the American Fertility Society 1990 Ethical considerations of the new reproductive technologies. *Fertility and Sterility* **53**(6):1–103

Garner GH 1985 Pregnancy after infertility. *Journal of Obstetric, Gynaecologic and Neonatal Nursing* **11**:58–62

Ghazi HA, Spielberger C, Kallan B 1991 Delivery outcome after infertility: a registry study. *Fertility and Sterility* **55**(4):726–32

Golombok S 1992 Psychological functioning in infertility patients. *Human Reproduction* **7**(2):208–12

Golombok S, Cook R, Bish A, Murray C 1995 Families created by the new reproductive technologies: quality of parenting and social and emotional development of the children. *Child Development* **66**:285–98

Goode CJ, Hahn SJ 1993 Oocyte donation and in vitro fertilisation: the nurse's role with ethical and legal issues. *Journal of Obstetric, Gynaecologic and Neonatal Nursing* **22**(2):106–11

Hargreaves Pearson L 1992 The stigma of infertility. *Nursing Times* **88**(1):36–8

Hodgkinson E 1992 *Counselling*. London: Simon & Schuster

Howie PW 1990 Selective reduction? Medical aspects. In Templeton A, Cuisine D (eds) *Reproductive Medicine and The Law*. Edinburgh: Churchill Livingstone

Human Fertilisation and Embryology Authority (HFEA) 1994 *Third Annual Report*. London: HFEA

Jones M 1991 *Infertility: Modern treatments and the issues they raise*. London: Judy Platous

Katz Rothman B 1988 *The Tentative Pregnancy*. London: Pandora Press

Kitzinger S 1978 *Women as Mothers*. Oxford: Fontana Books

Klein R 1989 Resistance. In Klein R (ed.) *Women Speak Out*. London: Pandora Press

Kon A 1993 Infertility – The Costs. A Report commissioned by ISSUE and CHILD

Kozolanka K 1989 Giving up the chance that isn't. In Klein R (ed.) *Women Speak Out*. London: Pandora Press

Kumar R 1982 Neurotic disorders in childbearing women. In Brockington IF, Kumar R (eds) *Motherhood and Mental Illness*. London: Academic Press

Lasker J, Borg S 1989 *In Search of Parenthood: Coping with infertility and high tech conception*. London: Pandora Press

MacFarlane AJ, Price F, Bryan F, Botting AJ 1990 *Three, Four or More. A Study of Triplet and Higher Order Births*. London: HMSO

Mahlstedt PP 1985 The psychological component of infertility. *Fertility and Sterility* **43**(3):313–19

Medical Research Council Working Party on Children Conceived by In Vitro Fertilisation 1990 Births in Great Britain resulting from assisted conception 1978–87. *British Medical Journal* **300**:1229–33

Morgan D, Lee RG 1991 *Blackstone's Guide to the Human Fertilisation and Embryology Act 1990*. London: Blackstone Press

Mushin D, Barreda-Hansom M, Spensley J 1986 I.V.F. children – early psychological development. *Journal of In Vitro Fertilisation and Embryo Transfer* **14**:247–52

Oakley A 1986 *Subject Women*. London: Fontana

O'Donovan K 1990 What shall we tell the children? In Lee R, Morgan D (eds) *Birthrights: Law and ethics at the beginning of life*. London: Routledge

Pappert A 1989 A Voice for Infertile Women. In Klein R (ed.) *Women Speak Out*. London: Pandora Press

Price F 1990 Establishing guidelines: regulation and the clinical management of infertility. In Lee R, Morgan D (eds) *Birthrights: Law and ethics at the beginning of life*. London: Routledge

Raphael-Leff J 1991 *Psychological Processes of Childbearing*. London: Chapman & Hall

Ravel H, Slade P, Buck P. Lieberman B 1987 The impact of infertility on emotions and the marital and sexual relationship. *Journal of Reproductive and Infant Psychology* **5**:221–34

Reid S 1988 *Labour of Love: The story of the world's first surrogate grandmother*. London: Bodley Head

Rubin R 1984 *Maternal Identity and the Maternal Experience*. New York: Springer

Rufat P, Oliviennes F, Mouzon J, Dehan M, Frydman R 1994 Task force report on the outcome of pregnancies and children conceived by in vitro fertilisation (France 1987–1989). *Fertility and Sterility* **61**(2):324–30

Silverton L 1993 The elderly primagravida. In Alexander J, Levy V, Roch S (eds) *Midwifery Practice: A research-based approach*. Basingstoke: Macmillan

Snowden R 1984 *The Gift of a Child*. London: Allen & Unwin

Toynbee P 1985 *Lost Children*. London: Hutchinson

Warnock M 1992 *A Question of Life*. Oxford: Blackwell

Winkler U 1989 He called me Number 27. In Klein R (ed.) *Women Speak Out*. London: Pandora Press

Winston R 1987 *Infertility: A sympathetic approach*. London: Martin Durity

Woollett A 1989 Commentary articles, special issue on Psychology and Infertility. *Journal of Reproductive and Infant Psychology* 1991 **9**:49–59

Wood C, Westmore A 1984 *Test Tube Conception*. London: George Allen & Unwin

Yovich J, Parry T, French N, Gravang A 1986 Developmental assessment of twenty I.V.F. infants at their first birthday. *Journal of In Vitro Fertilisation and Embryo Transfer* **3**:253–7

FURTHER READING

Bryan E 1992 *Twins and Higher Order Multiple Births: A guide to their nature and nurture*. London: Edward Arnold

Jennings SE 1995 *Infertility Counselling*. Oxford: Blackwell Scientific

Meerabeau L, Denton J 1996 *Infertility, Nursing and Caring*. London: Scutari Press

USEFUL ADDRESSES

British Infertility Counselling Association
69 Bibision Street
Sheffield S1 4GE

CHILD
Charter House
43 St Leonards Road
Bexhill-on-Sea
East Sussex TN40 1JA   Tel: 01424 732361

Provides information, counselling and support to infertile couples.

Human Fertilisation and Embryology Authority
Paxton House
30 Artillery Lane
London E1 7LS   Tel: 0171-377 5077
                                 Fax: 0171-377 1871

ISSUE (The National Fertility Association)
509 Aldridge Road
Great Barr
Birmingham B44 8NA   Tel: 0121-344 4414
                                 Fax: 0121-344 4336

Provides continuing help for people experiencing difficulty in conception.

TAMBA (The Twins and Multiple Births Association)
59 Sunnyside
Worksop
Notts. S81 7LN   Tel: (01909) 479250

Supports families with twins, triplets or more through a network of over
200 Twins Clubs throughout the UK. Promotes understanding among the
public and medical and education professions of the needs of such families.
Specialist support groups for parents of 'supertwins' (three or more) with
special needs. The Health and Education Group provides a parents–professional partnership. Students' packs and speakers are available.

CHAPTER TEN

Drug misuse and pregnancy

Catherine Siney

Pregnant women with a history of drug misuse present midwives with a particular set of challenges. This chapter explores these and suggests some strategies for responding to them.

Most of us indulge in some degree of drug use – the comforting cup of coffee, the sociable alcoholic drink, the welcome cigarette – so it is important to define exactly what is meant by the terms 'drug misuse', 'drug dependence' and 'problem drug taker'.

The Department of Health (1991) defines 'drug misuse' as:

'drug taking which is hazardous or harmful and unsanctioned by professional or cultural standards. It is broadly equivalent to terms such as 'drug abuse' and 'problem drug taking'.

The Department of Health (1991) definition of 'drug dependence' is:

the altered physical and psychological state which results in disturbed physical and mental functioning when the drug is abruptly discontinued. It is broadly equivalent to 'addiction'. Not all drug misusers are drug dependent.

The United Kingdom Advisory Council on the Misuse of Drugs (1982) definition of the problem drug taker is:

any person who experiences social, psychological, physical or legal problems related to intoxication and/or regular excessive consumption and/or dependence as a consequence of his/her own use of drugs or chemical substances.

Pregnancy in female drug misusers has been a recognised phenomenon since the mid 1980s. However, there has been little change in the midwifery/obstetric management of these women in the UK (Fraser 1983; Kroll 1986; Gerada *et al.* 1990; Siney 1995). This is probably due to the lack of large-scale, up to date research in the care of pregnant drug users, which is in turn due to the failure of maternity services to identify the women concerned (Gerada *et al.* 1990). While pregnant drug users are regarded as a 'high-risk' obstetric group (Siney 1995), responding to their needs in the context of hospital antenatal care, or indeed any antenatal care, has proved a particular challenge.

HIV and AIDS in relation to drug misuse is not discussed in this chapter, being too large a subject to address only in part. It is to be hoped, however, that all clinical midwifery practice is based on an awareness of the high-risk potential of all body fluids from all women.

A WOMAN-CENTRED SERVICE

Following work undertaken in Liverpool (an area nationally acknowl-edged to have a large number of drug misusers, particularly opiate users), a midwife-led system of care was designed in an attempt to make both maternity and gynaecology in general, and antenatal services in partic-ular, more 'woman-centred' and therefore 'user friendly'.

The system was audited after the first year and a case–control study completed in 1993 (Siney *et al.* 1995). The care provided now enables women to look forward to their baby's birth with a level of optimism comparable to that enjoyed by non-drug-using women. Countrywide, however, there are different approaches to the care of pregnant women who use illegal drugs. It would appear that some women fear that they might encounter punitive or judgemental behaviour from midwifery and obstetric staff.

While it is accepted that any regular drug use (whether illicit or prescribed) during pregnancy will place a woman in a 'high-risk' category, a system of care that allows a woman to receive antenatal care in a relaxed way, allowing her to be open about her drug use, will enable health care providers to give her appropriate advice and build up a basis of knowledge about this largely hidden problem.

Identifying the client group

Doctors are obliged by law to notify the Addicts Index at the Home Office of contact with anyone they consider to be, or have reasonable grounds to suspect of being, addicted to controlled drugs. They should also report details of these patients to the appropriate Regional Drug Misuse Database. Compulsory admission to hospital under the Mental Health Act may be justified for a drug misuser who is also suffering from mental disorder, but drug misuse alone is not sufficient grounds for this.

An accurate estimate of the number of women of childbearing age in the UK is difficult to gauge. Drug misuse affects males and females equally, but patterns of drug use differ between the sexes. The availability of treat-ment programmes varies throughout the UK but, where programmes are available, they generally give pregnant women priority of access.

Because most drug services are geared to opiate users, there is a problem in identifying users of other drugs, such as cocaine. Cocaine is becoming an increasing problem in the UK, but the challenge it presents to the midwifery and obstetric services has much in common with that posed by other drugs. The best way to encourage both registered and non-registered drug users to identify themselves and attend for antenatal care is to develop an attractive woman-centred and non-judgemental service that guarantees confidentiality.

In some areas, midwifery and obstetric services have no information about known or registered drug misusers. A survey of obstetric units in England and Wales that asked for the actual or estimated number of babies born to drug-dependent women in the previous year, and compared that number with the number of drug-using women identified to regional databases, indicated that there were probably a large number of women not being identified (Morrison & Siney 1995). There are, of course, some areas where this is not the case.

A persuasive reason for midwives to identify which of the women in their caseload use drugs is to avoid them becoming even more marginalised by turning up 'unbooked' at delivery time. Early identification may also make paediatric problems in the postnatal period easier to deal with. Moreover, it is part of the midwifery challenge to ensure that women who might be considered to be 'high risk', and who might not be comfortable attending hospital or GP antenatal clinics, should have some antenatal care in a setting in which they feel at ease.

Another important clinical reason for identifying drug misusers who are pregnant is to ensure that they are aware of the risks of sudden opiate withdrawal. Cocaine and other stimulants can be stopped immediately without ill effects. If a pregnant woman uses opiates, however, her baby can suffer acute withdrawal symptoms, which may cause distress, may precipitate labour and may even be fatal. If an opiate-dependent woman wishes either to reduce or to stop using drugs, this should be done in a controlled manner. This can be achieved on either an inpatient or an outpatient basis.

There are many reasons why women do not identify themselves as drug misusers, the main one being that the attitudes of many people, particularly those involved in child care, towards drug misusers can be perceived to be judgemental. Consequently, women may fear that the professionals will assume that they will make bad mothers. According to the Department of Health (1991), being a drug user does not preclude the presence of parenting skills and is not necessarily a reason to separate mother and child. Any changes in attitude, however, are not universal.

Another reason why women do not identify themselves as drug users may be that they fear they will be treated differently from other pregnant or newly delivered women while in hospital. Such differences in treatment will probably be on the grounds that they will automatically be considered to be at higher risk from bloodborne infections (particularly HIV and hepatitis B and C) than the general public who do not admit to drug misuse or high-risk sexual behaviour.

Apart from the women's confidentiality and dignity, the risks to staff of being selective about the way they apply stringent principles of infection control cannot be overemphasised. All body fluids from all women should be considered to be risky to staff, and therefore clinical practices should be of the highest standard in every case and not just where a woman is known to be HIV positive or an intravenous drug user.

Trust is essential

It is important to build up trust, not only between women and those who work in the maternity services, but also between all professionals who work with drug-misusing women. This is equally true in areas where there are no statutory drug services. It is important that the women know that they will be cared for as other women are, and that they will not encounter adverse discrimination. Pregnant women who are comfortable about discussing their drug use with midwives enable the development of a real partnership in care. Always providing that confidentiality is not infringed, the expertise gained by the midwife and the outcomes of the pregnancies can then be shared with all agencies, both statutory and non-statutory. The more such sharing and interaction is possible, the more accurate information about the effects of drugs on pregnancy and the neonate will become available and can be given to drug users before they become pregnant.

THE LIVERPOOL EXPERIENCE

Attitudes can be positive or negative. Starting with the hypothesis that a supportive staff attitude would be most helpful to the client group, some drug awareness study days were set up in Liverpool as an initial step. Managerial, medical, nursing and social work staff from the local statutory drug service were invited to talk to the hospital and community staff. Information was given about drugs and treatment programmes, prescription of an opiate substitute (methadone) both in pregnancy and in general, and about drug misuse/dependency and childcare issues. The study days were popular and well attended. Following on from them, regular updating lectures are held during each year, and all grades of staff (both professional and ancillary) are welcome.

There was initially some resistance to the outreach work following in the wake of the study days, but this was overcome by the fact that although more drug misusers were identified as a result of it, the majority in reality caused no extra work or problems for the staff. There is now a simple management guideline in place.

A specialist midwife liaises with all services who work with drug misusers, be they statutory or non-statutory. Information that helps the drug-using woman to go through the maternity services is exchanged, with her knowledge. Any woman who admits drug misuse at any time is referred to the specialist midwife.

It is important for women to feel that they can talk truthfully at ante-natal interviews. The word 'use' instead of 'take' in relation to drugs is recognised by a drug user but will probably mean nothing to a non-drug user. By the language they speak, staff can indicate a non-judgemental attitude. This in turn enables the women to ask questions about the effects of drug use on their fetus and allows staff to explain the principles that will be followed in the planning of maternity care and the care of the newborn child.

A woman who is on a controlled programme of opiate withdrawal and receiving a regular methadone (opiate substitute) prescription is likely to see herself no longer as an addict. People in this situation may refer to the methadone as 'medicine' and can easily be offended if this is forgotten.

Access to systems of care

In Liverpool, referrals are made to the specialist midwife from drug services and GPs who prescribe methadone to their patients, and the probation service and social services; women also self-refer. Antenatal care and advice is offered freely to women whether or not they are registered for treatment, and whether or not they are booked into a hospital for the birth. If the women want to deliver their babies at the Liverpool Women's Hospital, they can be booked by the specialist midwife wherever she sees them. Antenatal visits should be arranged at least monthly at any site, including drug clinics, GP surgeries and the hospital. No extra visits to hospital are required purely because of drug addiction. When attending hospital, the women are seen wherever possible by the same senior doctor (either consultant or senior registrar), thus giving some continuity of obstetric care.

The hospital pharmacy is kept up to date with accurate information about the amount of methadone prescribed and its approximate equiva-lent in 'street opiates' for women who are not 'notified' drug users. This should enable a guaranteed supply of methadone for all women who are admitted to hospital.

In Liverpool, a guideline for the treatment and care of infants of drug misusers has been designed, together with a non-subjective neonatal opiate withdrawal chart (Figure 10.1).

Figure 10.1   *Neonatal drug withdrawal chart*

Name: _____ **Casenote No:** _____ **D.O.B.:** _____ **Gestation:** _____

All infants of drug misusers must have observations started from birth.
Observations made post-feed.
Severe symptoms – please tick (✓) if present.

Date:										
Time:										
1. Convulsions										
2. Tremors when undisturbed. Non-stop high pitched cry. Sleeps < 1 h after good feed. (All must be present to score)										
3. Watery stools or projectile vomiting or requirement of tube feeds.										
Signature:										

Date:										
Time:										
1. Convulsions										
2. Tremors when undisturbed. Non-stop high pitched cry. Sleeps < 1 h after good feed. (All must be present to score)										
3. Watery stools or projectile vomiting or requirement of tube feeds.										
Signature:										

Date:										
Time:										
1. Convulsions										
2. Tremors when undisturbed. Non-stop high pitched cry. Sleeps < 1 h after good feed. (All must be present to score)										
3. Watery stools or projectile vomiting or requirement of tube feeds.										
Signature:										

Instructions for Treatment

Minor symptoms **need not** be recorded. These may include:

* *Tremors when disturbed   *Respiration > 60 per minute,
* *Pyrexia of unknown origin,   *Sweating,
* *Frequent yawning   *Sneezing/nasal stuffiness,
* *Poor feeding/regurgitation   *Loose stools.

If treatment of any of the 3 **severe** symptoms is not judged clinically necessary, then reasons must be recorded in casenotes.

Treatment:
Dose:
0.04 mg/kg morphine sulphate orally, every 4 hours.
Commence treatment 4 hourly ('treatment level5'). Then reduce the level of treatment every 24 hours as follows if severe symptoms are not present:

        0.04mg/kg morphine sulphate 6 hourly   ('treatment level 4')
        0.04mg/kg morphine sulphate 8 hourly   ('treatment level 3')
        0.04mg/kg morphine sulphate 12 hourly   ('treatment level 2')
        0.04mg/kg morphine sulphate daily   ('treatment level 1')

If severe symptoms persist, do not reduce the level of treatment

If severe symptoms persist on 4 hourly morphine ('treatment level 5') discuss, with a senior paediatrician, the possibility of increasing the dose of morphine or adding other medication.

The intention of these is to make it easy for the midwife to monitor the baby whatever her experience of drug misuse. This enables the mother to see that there can be no bias in monitoring and also ensures that babies who require treatment are treated both when necessary and appropriately. There is no difference in the quality of care received by drug-using (compared with non-drug-using) mothers, either during labour or in the postnatal period. Nor are the drug-using mothers and their babies cared for separately from either each other or others. This egalitarian approach maximises the likelihood of the woman's privacy, dignity and confidentiality being maintained while she is in hospital.

Regular, informal antenatal meetings are held with the senior hospital social worker, the liaison health visitor and the specialist liaison midwife, which include input from any key workers. This has made it possible to develop a discharge policy that can be discussed with the women during the course of the pregnancy. If there are no statutory reasons for a child protection conference, and mother and baby are both medically fit, they are transferred to community midwifery care following paediatric review 72 to 96 hours after delivery. If required, statutory child protection conferences are arranged before delivery so that the women's admission to, and transfer from, hospital can be as well organised as possible.

The maternity service for drug users would not be possible without the support of all agencies involved in the care of female drug misusers. Although the specialist drug liaison midwife is funded from obstetric resources, the support and information provision from other services is essential to the provision of optimum antenatal care.

Audit

It became obvious by the uptake that the service provided in Liverpool was popular with drug misusers. However, some form of audit was needed to measure the system of care that had evolved and its outcome for the women involved.

The resultant case–control study considered the care and progress of over 100 women. All of these were on a methadone programme with or without other drugs, all had received regular antenatal care and all had delivered in the unit during a 2-year period. The study, which is described in more detail elsewhere (Siney *et al.* 1995), aimed to test the hypothesis that regular antenatal care and a controlled methadone prescription minimised the risks incurred by opiate-dependent women and their babies, in comparison with their non-drug-using counterparts.

The results of the study confirmed the hypothesis. There was no infant or maternal mortality and no infant morbidity attributable to drug misuse. However, two babies born to drug-using mothers had congenital malformations – one a cleft lip and palate, and one severe hydrocephalus that had been diagnosed before birth. There were fewer antenatal admissions in the case group than in the control group, and babies were admitted to the neonatal intensive care unit only if there was a specific medical need. All monitoring of babies for opiate withdrawal signs was carried out on the wards using the neonatal opiate withdrawal chart (Figure 10.1).

These findings reinforce the claims made by Broekhuizen *et al.* (1992) that risks could be minimised if women taking opiate drugs could only be identified and given appropriate care and support during pregnancy. However, the study also highlighted some features that might be attributable to drug use itself rather that to the (often associated) economic deprivation. Despite outreach and an effort to provide a 'woman-centred' service, late booking with the maternity services was common – over half the women did not present themselves for antenatal care until well into the second trimester. While this may reflect a reluctance to seek care, it may also be due in part to the menstrual irregularities associated with opiate dependence (Morrison *et al.* 1995).

The higher incidence of low birthweight might be due to illegal drug use, but the results of the study were more suggestive of cigarette smoking as the main causative factor (Siney *et al.* 1995). The increased incidence of preterm delivery was consistent with earlier findings (Klenka 1986) and could have been associated with a greater incidence of infection in drug-using mothers (Marx *et al.* 1991; Lamont & Fisk 1992).

The results of this study underpin the guidance for antenatal, intrapartum and postnatal care of mothers and babies, and also the administration of methadone, in the Liverpool Women's Hospital.

GUIDELINES FOR MIDWIVES

Guidance on the management of pregnant substance abusers

The following is adapted from the guidance drawn up by the Liverpool Women's Hospital and following the results of the Liverpool research (Siney *et al.* 1995).

1. The aim of the management should be to 'normalise' as much as possible. All substance abusers are known by or notified to the drug liaison specialist midwife. The specialist midwife is notified by the prescribing agency (or GP) or directly by the records clerks or the midwives/doctors at booking. Some unregistered women may be known only to her.
2. All known substance abusers are booked under a named consultant. The specialist midwife can book direct to the consultant.
3. Care may be shared with the GP, the specialist midwife or both. Uptake of antenatal care is expected at least monthly.

4. Some women may see only the specialist midwife. If the women are booked in drug clinics, 'drop-ins' or at home, the specialist midwife will arrange for an ultrasound scan and a hospital appointment. The specialist midwife sees substance abusers at least monthly throughout pregnancy if they are not attending antenatal services elsewhere.

5. Registered misusers may receive methadone from drug clinics, GPs, the probation services or the local Drugs Council. The methadone regime advised by the drug prescribing units is stabilisation in the first trimester, reduction (if possible) in the second trimester, by a maximum of 5 mg per week, and maintenance in the third trimester. GPs may decide not to follow this prescribing regime. Some women do reduce intake up to the end of the pregnancy, but this should only be tried if they are stable. It is better not to reduce methadone if they are going to increase heroin. Stability should be encouraged, and neonatal withdrawal symptoms and any treatment for the baby explained.

6. Advice concerning prescribing for unregistered drug users may be obtained during office hours from the local drug dependency unit.

7. The risk from unmonitored or sudden drug withdrawal either in pregnancy or during labour should be explained; stability is more useful. Not only may withdrawal cause the fetus to become distressed, but opiate withdrawal may also make the uterus irritable, thus disguising early or premature labour. It may also precipitate labour.

8. All drug misusers are routinely offered a blood test for hepatitis B and C (HBsAg, Anti-HBc and Anti-HCV should be specifically requested on the test request form). HIV testing is not offered, and drug users who request HIV testing should be referred to the relevant drugs agency (the specialist midwife should have details of this). Most units also have an HIV testing protocol. Urine may only be tested for drugs if the woman gives permission.

9. During labour, methadone is given as prescribed, *together* with any analgesia required. Methadone is prescribed as a daily dose while drug-using women are inpatients. It can be asked for at any time and in a split dose over the 24 hours; women might not ask for all they have been prescribed.

10. The hospital pharmacy should hold a list of methadone users. This list, which should be updated regularly, should also indicate the amount of methadone each person is prescribed and the name of the prescriber. Pharmacy guidelines should be available on each ward/department. Part of the specialist midwife's responsibility is to tell the pharmacy of non-registered opiate addicts and, if it is known, the approximate amount of opiate used.

11. Withdrawal of opiates in labour may be seen as fetal distress on the CTG monitor. It is therefore helpful to ensure that the woman has an adequate amount of methadone throughout labour, so that the opiate withdrawal-induced fetal distress can be excluded from a list of possible obstetric emergencies.

12. The Unit's own research, comparing 103 treated opiate users with controls (Siney *et al.* 1995), has shown that opiate users in labour use 'normal' amounts of analgesia provided that methadone levels are maintained. Unregistered (i.e. untreated) opiate users will usually require larger amounts of opiates for pain relief in labour, unless methadone is given to stabilise their withdrawal.

13. Mothers and babies are kept together and use any bed in the postnatal area. No isolation and no special infection control procedures are required.

14. Discharge is after 72 to 96 hours because of research findings demonstrating that neonatal withdrawal symptoms from methadone (which has a longer half-life than heroin) generally occur (if at all) after 24 hours. If they have not occurred by 72 hours, or if they begin to occur in mild form at that stage, there is generally no problem after discharge (Siney *et al.* 1995). Babies who show no symptoms of opiate withdrawal postnatally have often shown fetal distress *in utero* during labour, often requiring instrumental or operative delivery. Babies with severe symptoms are treated as indicated in Figure 10.1. If mothers are also using benzodiazepines, an extra day is required before review.

15. All substance misusers known to the specialist midwife are reviewed regularly by her, the senior hospital social workers and the health visitor liaison. The need for formal social service input will be decided by them before the birth.

Management of infants of substance abusers

This is adapted from the guidelines drawn up by the Liverpool Women's Hospital and following the results of the Liverpool research (Siney *et al.* 1995).

1. Where a pregnant woman is a known 'substance abuser' (heroin, alcohol, barbiturates, etc.), the midwives or doctors will alert the drug liaison midwife (DLM). The DLM will then inform the relevant agencies and personnel. Urine from a woman who is suspected of drug abuse can only be tested for this with her consent.

2. At birth, a paediatric SHO will attend, and the infant's condition, weight, etc. will be assessed. The paediatric SHO should be informed of

delivery. The social worker must be informed by the ward staff if he or she is involved in the woman's care.

3. Infants of 'substance abusers' should be nursed on the ward with their mother, unless there are medical indications for admission to SCBU. These include major convulsions and birth asphyxia.

4. Severely symptomatic infants of opiate users are treated as outlined in Figure 10.1.

5. Severe signs of withdrawal are generalised convulsions, tremors when undisturbed, a continuous high-pitched cry, sleeping for less than 1 hour after feeding, projectile vomiting, watery stools and a hyperactive Moro reflex.

6. Mild signs of withdrawal include sneezing, frequent yawning, tremors when disturbed, poor feeding, sleeping for less than 3 hours after feeding, respiration rate greater than 60 per minute, sweating, regurgitation, raised temperature, excoriation of the nose, knees or toes, loose stools and nasal stuffiness.

7. The social work department will determine the need for a case conference, informal review, follow-up or supervision with relevant agencies.

8. Discharge is after review at 72 to 96 hours if there are no medical problems. Babies may have mild symptoms on discharge.

Pointers for practice

1. Is there any way to establish links with the drug services in your area in order to see whether there is a service need?

2. Does identification of drug misuse in a pregnant woman mean notification of district social services department and a child protection conference? Does this affect whether mothers identify themselves?

3. Are known or suspected drug misusers automatically offered testing for hepatitis B and C and/or HIV? Are pretest counselling and support available?

4. Are extra or different infection control procedures used for known drug misusers? Does this breach confidentiality?

5. Are babies of known drug misusers separated from their mothers and cared for elsewhere? If so, why? Does it affect whether mothers identify themselves?

6. If your hospital uses a neonatal withdrawal chart, is it a subjective one? What if a midwife has never before cared for the baby of a drug-using mother?

7. Are the expectations of baby care in the postnatal period higher for known drug misusers than for non-drug users?

Conclusion

Drug use in pregnancy is associated with many problems and, even in Liverpool where concerted efforts have been made, by no means all of these have been solved. A number of unregistered women still turn up 'unbooked' in labour (although only one in 1995). The Liverpool approach, however, has considerably contributed towards the improvement of services to this particular group of vulnerable women (Siney *et al.* 1995) and the underlying system of care with others. This service relies very much on non-technological aspects. Indications are that the only way to encourage both registered and non-registered drug users to identify and attend for antenatal care is to develop an attractive, low-key, woman-centred service that guarantees confidentiality and sympathetic care.

This chapter has concentrated on drugs of physical dependence, i.e opioids, because the maternal dependence, which causes the neonatal dependence, is what leads to the problems and risks. Opioids are, however, not the only drugs that are misused, and the majority of dependent women will probably be using other drugs too, for example, benzodiazepines (usually temazepam and diazepam) amphetamines, cocaine (usually in the form of 'crack'), cannabis and occasionally Ecstasy, although the latter is generally stopped when women realise that they are pregnant.

Other variables that should be considered are cigarette smoking and alcohol use (Plant 1990) and poverty or deprivation (see Chapter 4 in this volume). All of these, even without the use of illegal substances, can affect the outcome of pregnancy.

Acknowledgements

Thanks are due to Mr Steve Walkinshaw, Mr Mervyn Kidd and all staff at Liverpool Women's Hospital; also to Dr Clive Morrison, Dr Sue Ruben, all staff at the Liverpool Drug Dependency Clinic and all staff within Liverpool and surrounding Drug Services, both statutory and non-statutory.

REFERENCES

Broekhuizen FF, Utrie J, Van Mullem C 1992 Drug use or inadequate prenatal care? Adverse pregnancy outcome in an urban setting. *American Journal of Obstetrics and Gynecology* **166**(6):1747–56

Department of Health 1991 *Drug Misuse and Dependence. Guidelines on Clinical Management.* London: HMSO

Fraser AC 1983 The pregnant drug addict. *Maternal and Child Health* Nov: 461–3

Gerada C, Dawe S, Farrell M 1990 Management of the pregnant opiate user. *British Journal of Hospital Medicine* **43**:138–41

Klenka HM 1986 Babies born in a district general hospital to mothers taking heroin. *British Medical Journal* **298**:745–6

Kroll D 1986 Heroin addiction in pregnancy. *Midwives Chronicle and Nursing Notes* **99** (1182):153–7

Lamont RF, Fisk N 1992 The role of infection in the pathogenesis of preterm labour. *Progress in Obstetrics and Gynaecology* **10**:135–58

Marx R, Aral SO, Rolfs RT, Sterk CE, Kahn JG 1991 Crack, sex and STD. *Sexually Transmitted Diseases* **18**:92–101

Morrison C, Siney C 1995 Maternity services for drug misusers in England and Wales: a national survey. *Health Trends* **27**(1)

Morrison CL, Ruben SM, Beeching NJ 1995 Female sexual health problems in a drug dependency clinic. *International Journal of STD and AIDS* **6**:201–3

Plant M 1990 Maternal alcohol and tobacco use during pregnancy. In Alexander J, Levy V, Roch S (eds) *Antenatal Care: A research-based approach*. Basingstoke: Macmillan

Siney C 1995 Drug abusing mothers. In Alexander J, Levy V, Roch S (eds) *Aspects of Midwifery Practice: A research-based approach*. Basingstoke: Macmillan

Siney C, Kidd M, Walkinshaw S, Morrison C, Manasse P 1995 Opiate dependency in pregnancy. *British Journal of Midwifery* **3**(2):69–73

United Kingdom Advisory Council on the Misuse of Drugs (UKACMD) 1992 *Treatment and Rehabilitation*. London: HMSO

FURTHER READING

Department of Health 1991 *Drug Misuse and Dependence. Guidelines on Clinical Management*. London: HMSO

Institute for the Study of Drug Dependence 1992 *Drugs, Pregnancy and Childcare. A Guide for Professionals*. London: ISDD

Siney C, Kidd M, Walkinshaw S, Morrison C, Manasse P 1995 Opiate dependency in pregnancy. *British Journal of Midwifery* **3**(2):69–73

Siney C (ed.) 1995 *The Pregnant Drug Addict*. Manchester: Books for Midwives Press

United Kingdom Advisory Council on the Misuse of Drugs 1992 *Treatment and Rehabilitation*. London: HMSO

CHAPTER ELEVEN

Multiple sclerosis and midwifery care

Meg Taylor

INTRODUCTION

For most women, adjusting to pregnancy and motherhood is a challenging experience. Although birth is usually an optimistic and enriching experience, it is not without difficulties and traumas. For women contemplating motherhood who also have a disability such as multiple sclerosis (MS), the journey can be especially difficult. There are sometimes problems in providing sensitive women-centred care for women with disabilities, and these problems may stem from misunderstandings, lack of knowledge and inappropriate attitudes based on stereotypical images of women and disabled people. Midwives and other carers involved in caring for women in childbirth sometimes need to be helped to see the 'normal mother' inside the disabled woman. When this happens the woman can be helped to grow in confidence and competence.

To be pregnant and disabled presents women with the double disadvantage of being female in a world dominated by a male-dominated medical model of care, and negative attitudes towards disability and handicap. To able-bodied midwives and other carers who often cannot see beyond the disability, signs and symptoms such as impaired mobility may seem to be the only issue worthy of consideration and concern. Negative and myopic attitudes from those who offer care may make a complex situation even worse. Midwives are sometimes afraid to, or refuse to, confront the facts and implications of disability, perhaps hoping that if it is ignored it will go away. This often means that the environment is unnecessarily difficult and inaccessible.

These negative attitudes often include a belief that disability implies low intelligence, that it is the same as illness, that disabled people must be dependent on the able bodied, or that a disabled person is somehow not a proper person. More specifically, with regard to childbirth, there may be an unspoken assumption that people with disabilities should not reproduce. There may be distaste or embarrassment that disabled people are sexually active and attractive, and there may be an automatic assumption that a woman with a disability will need a caesarean section and that the child is at risk. These attitudes exist in a context where there are few if any positive images in the media of people with disabilities and where there is a general awkwardness and embarrassment in the presence of disabled people.

According to Campion (1990), neither being pregnant nor being disabled is an illness, and therefore the expertise for either cannot rest solely with the medical profession. MS is the most common disorder of the central nervous system (CNS) in the UK, and the treatment and care of childbearing women with this condition require the help and support of a multidisciplinary team that might include midwives, obstetricians and neurologists as well as those in the professions allied to medicine.

MS results from episodes of neuritis that cause permanent damage to the myelin, which is the fatty sheath surrounding certain nerves in the CNS. In a healthy state, this sheath improves the efficiency of nerve impulse transmission. 'Sclerosis' refers to the hardened areas or plaques that cover these areas of damage or demyelination, and 'multiple' refers to both the number and location of lesions. Lesions may occur in any part of the CNS and with varying frequency. For this reason, MS is unpredictable and idiosyncratic. Each sufferer will have a unique experience of MS, and lesions may cause a variety of symptoms. These can include visual disturbances, leading in rare cases to blindness, numbness and tingling of the limbs, a sensation of weakness, which may or may not impair movement, spasticity, incontinence of urine, urgency of micturition, impotence in men and loss of sexual sensation in women, inappropriate sensations of heat or cold, and many other symptoms. The degree of impairment experienced by people with MS can vary considerably. In some instances, there are no symptoms, MS only being diagnosed at post mortem and when death has occurred for a quite different reason. In others there is a steady and inevitable decline in function leading to total dependence, death being caused by an opportunistic infection.

MS AND MIDWIFERY CARE

MS is of relevance to midwives for two reasons: women are diagnosed more often than men, in a ratio of 2:1, and the age of diagnosis reaches its peak in the thirties, a time when women are still of reproductive age. However, MS is more than just a physical condition: it is a condition with complex physical, psychological and social components that interweave in a complex way and may mutually influence the course of the condition. Orthodox medicine sees MS primarily and totally as a physical condition, but the experience of someone with MS may involve considerably more than this. To exclude the emotional, psychological and spiritual aspects of care is a mistake. The physical effects of the condition are only one aspect, and the midwife must consider the woman and her needs in total. For example, to the newly pregnant women who also has MS, living with despair and the grief for the loss of an apparently 'normal' life may be more crippling than her physical symptoms. The effects of social stigmatisation and insensitive social policies that ignore the needs of the disabled are also likely to have a detrimental effect on the quality of life of the woman and her family. These are some of the reasons why MS may be described not only as a physical illness, but also as a psychological or social disorder. This is confirmed in a British Society of Rehabilitation Medicine study (BSRM 1993), which reports that 90 per cent of those questioned described themselves as handicapped even though 1 in 3 of those with MS interviewed showed no sign of physical handicap. It would appear that the experience of MS can be more debilitating than physical signs alone would suggest.

THE CAUSE AND NATURE OF MS

The condition of MS seems even to confuse the charitable organisation established to support those with this illness. The MS Society's advertisements paint a stark black and white picture of MS in terms of dependency and impairment. They describe sufferers as needing someone to pick up the pieces and give them guidance. Words such as 'shattered' are used, and reference is made to blindness. 'Shattered' may indeed be the case as some women are exhausted by the emotional consequences of the condition, but for many it is not the physical symptoms that lead to the adverse emotional effects. According to the Society's own leaflets, 1 in 3 people with MS show no sign of physical disability and fewer than 1 in 5 will need a wheelchair.

The BSRM states that MS occurs in over 1 in 1000 of the UK population (BSRM 1993), but there is little evidence to support the negative stance taken in fundraising advertising literature. It is clear from the medical evidence of the condition that, given the unpredictable and idiosyncratic nature of MS, it is impossible to predict either the course or outcome of the condition. It is this feature that insists that midwives offer women with MS the benefits associated with carefully planned, thoughtful individualised care.

Matthews (1985) describes the typical course of the condition in the following way:

> A woman aged approximately thirty will experience an initial attack, most commonly of retrobulbar neuritis, numbness or weakness. She will make a complete recovery after some weeks. No diagnosis will be made at this point. After an interval which may vary from several months to several years she will experience a second attack, usually with different symptoms from the

first. Again she will make a complete recovery. She will have a further attack within the next couple of years which will usually be more severe and leave her often with permanent symptoms or a slight disability. This pattern continues for three to four years, each time with a slightly worse recovery. After about five years the pattern changes. There are no more complete attacks and recoveries, instead her symptoms fluctuate from day to day. This phase may last for years. If the disease is to become chronic and degenerative this phase will be followed by a progressive decline which in the worst cases will leave the sufferer bedridden and helpless. Memory and concentration will go, and death usually occurs as a result of pneumonia or kidney damage due to bladder paralysis. Conversely, if the condition is benign there will be no evident handicap.

MS has traditionally been described as two types: acute (relapsing with the better prognosis) and chronic (degenerative). MacAlpine's 'Multiple Sclerosis' (Matthews *et al.* 1991) uses three terms: remittent, remittent/progressive, and progressive from the outset. However, it is impossible to predict the course the illness will take in any individual, especially at the time of diagnosis, as this is usually made comparatively early in the course of the disorder.

THE GENERAL EFFECTS OF CHILDBEARING ON MS

There is some evidence that MS is affected by the female hormones oestrogen and progesterone. Some women experience worse symptoms in the premenstrual period (Matthews *et al.* 1991). However, the additional hormones of pregnancy seem, on the whole, to induce a feeling of well-being. Forti and Segal (undated) found the relapse rate in the first half of pregnancy to be the same as for a non-pregnant woman, but noted an improvement in the second half of pregnancy.

Women are at a greater risk of relapse in the postnatal period, but this increased risk seems to be compensated for by the reduced risk during pregnancy. Overall, the evidence suggests that childbearing has no adverse effect on the course of the condition, and indeed neurologists do not advise against pregnancy. In the sample of women examined by Forti and Segal, 40–50 per cent experienced relapses in the first 3–6 months following childbirth; of these 80 per cent recovered fully.

Some women report that their experience of their condition can fluctuate even from hour to hour, and not surprisingly some women find that some aspects of pregnancy, labour and the puerperium can lead to a deterioration in some symptoms of MS. For example, the altered carbohydrate metabolism of pregnancy, which often leads to a sense of increased hunger and can contribute to increased feelings of nausea, and the increased blood volume, which in turn increases sensitivity to heat, can also cause an exacerbation of a wide range of symptoms. Increasing weight and size can lead to problems with balance, which may worsen existing problems in this area. Pressure of the fetal head on the bladder can make urinary control more difficult. Fatigue may become worse, more unpredictable and difficult to control. Labour can be stressful, and stress can also influence the intensity of the symptoms in some women. In the postnatal period fatigue is often the major cause of symptoms; both the immediate fatigue following labour and the chronic fatigue resulting from broken nights' sleep contribute to a time of increased physical and psychological stress to a woman whose health is already compromised by MS. A raised temperature, due to either infection or breast engorgement, can also cause an exacerbation of symptoms.

It is especially important that midwives warn and advise women of these changes and explain that they often relate to pregnancy and are not necessarily due to a decline in the condition.

MS AND THE PROCESS OF CHILDBIRTH

Conception and preconception

According to Matthews *et al.* (1991), MS has no influence on fertility or the rate of spontaneous miscarriage. Forti and Segal (undated) suggest that the effects of MS may influence a woman's desire to conceive. They considered it likely that women with MS may have difficulties in accepting themselves as sexually active, and that their sense of themselves as disabled and abnormal may lead them to think that sex and childbearing are or should be out of the question. Some women with MS experience a reduced or absent sensation in the genital area, but while this has an obvious impact on the experience of sexual pleasure, it does not preclude conception. It is also possible that a woman with MS may want to have a child to demonstrate that, in that aspect of her life at least, she is normal.

However, many women with MS do not want to have children or reluctantly feel that they ought not to have children, or consider themselves physically incapable of caring for a child. Although Matthews *et al.* (1991) give no figures, they describe the rate of termination of pregnancy among women with MS as 'high'.

On the other hand, Campion (1990) defends the right of women with disabilities to have children if they so choose and outlines a series of questions such a woman might ask herself before conception:

How well adjusted do you think you are to your disability?

How active a life are you able to lead?

How much help do you require with daily tasks?

Is your disability likely to deteriorate in the future or result in a shorter life span? If so, is your partner able, and prepared, to take on the additional responsibilities of caring for a child?

Do you have a support network of friends and/or relatives nearby on whom you can call for support, both emotional and practical?

Have you any experience of looking after other people's children?

Do you foresee any major practical problems with looking after a child?

Do you live in accommodation that is suitable, or can be adapted, for you to look after a child?

Do you have a garden for messy play?

Are you reasonably secure financially?

Do you live in a community where you are known and where you know other people with young children? If not, would you consider moving?

Do you feel you would be a burden to your children? Is this a real possibility or a guilty worry?

Do you have a good relationship with your partner and would he be supportive?

Do you have confidence in your own ability to face the challenges that come with looking after a child?

These are generally sensible and practical questions for any woman contemplating a pregnancy but may be especially helpful for a woman with MS.

Heritability

The children of parents with MS are at increased risk of developing MS themselves. This increased risk varies according to the sex of the affected parent and the child. Because women are affected more than men, the daughter of a woman with MS is most at risk: her chance of developing MS is as high as 1 in 100 compared with 1 in 1000 for the general population (Forti and Segal undated). The risk for boys falls somewhere between these two figures.

Pregnancy

In some women, pregnancy is the time when MS can improve, at least temporarily, and it is possible for some symptoms to be milder or at least less frequent; for some, mobility can improve. For others pregnancy and childbirth may lead to a worsening of MS symptoms and an increased rate of relapse. However, the fact that a woman has MS does not mean that the wellbeing of her fetus will be compromised; MS does not necessarily indicate a high-risk pregnancy. Women who take drugs to ameliorate the condition must take special care before and during pregnancy and seek the specialist advice of their neurologist, pharmacist and obstetrician.

According to Fortis and Segal (undated), any drug should be discontinued, including those taken to stop spasm (for example baclofen, diazepam, dantrolene sodium), to control urinary frequency or incontinence (for example flavoxate hydrochloride) or long-term therapies such as azathioprine. These authors argue that because the risk of relapse is reduced, the need for steroids is also reduced. This is not, however, the established medical view, which is that stopping either anticonvulsants or steroids is dangerous. The prospect of pregnancy will necessitate a review of the medication prescribed for people with MS. Risks and benefits will be assessed for each drug. The abrupt withdrawal of some medications, such as anticonvulsants or corticosteroids, could prove dangerous.

The UK and US guidelines for some drugs commonly used in MS are set out in Figure 11.1, Figure 11.2 including more detail on US drug categories. Antenatal care of women taking anticonvulsants is outlined in Figure 11.3. Information on vitamins in pregnancy is summarised in Figure 11.4.

For a women with MS, the normal minor conditions of pregnancy can easily be confused with symptoms of MS. These symptoms include urinary frequency or stress incontinence, increased fatigue, constipation and reduced mobility due to increasing weight and size. These symptoms may be particularly distressing for a woman with MS, who may be perceived as unduly anxious.

To some extent most pregnant women experience episodes of acute and increased anxiety. Not least, the modern array of screening and diagnostic tests tend to promote rather than allay anxiety in the first instance. Pregnancy, like MS, is a condition in which uncertainty is intrinsic. Pregnant women with MS who are well used to uncertainty may weather the uncertainty of pregnancy especially well, but they may also experience some emotional turbulence. Any change in circumstances leads to loss, however small, and these losses can evoke past losses. It is possible that pregnancy can bring about a flashback of the grief that accompanied the diagnosis of MS, and the midwife should be alert and sensitive to seemingly irrational fears and concerns.

Figure 11.1 *Pregnancy and drugs used in MS*

Muscle relaxants

Baclofen   Toxicity (developmental and skeletal abnormalities) in the fetus in animal studies (BNF 1995). Safety in pregnancy not established. US category C (Karch 1992)

Diazepam   Toxicity in first trimester reported in some texts (Karch 1992; Medawar 1992). Risks of cardiac or gut defects, cleft palate, microcephaly in the first trimester. Neonatal withdrawal syndrome likely after prolonged use. Avoid during labour and delivery due to risk of 'floppy infant' syndrome (Malseed *et al.* 1995). US category D

Dantrolene   Safety not established. Little experience with this drug. US category C

Immunosuppressants

Azathioprine This crosses the placenta and has shown teratogenicity in animal studies. All patients are carefully monitored for marrow toxicity; the risks and consequences of infection during pregnancy should be borne in mind. Azathioprine therapy is rarely initiated during pregnancy. BNF (1995) advises that azathioprine has not proved teratogenic when used during pregnancy in renal transplant recipients. US category D

Corticosteroids Neonatal adrenal suppression is a known hazard, particularly with doses over 10 mg per day prednisolone, or equivalent, during the last two trimesters. Close supervision will be required to titrate dose against disease. Any dose adjustments must be made gradually under the guidance of the physician. The risks and benefits will be considered in each individual case. During labour, additional steroids will be required by the mother (BNF 1995). US category C

Anti-muscarinics

Flavoxate   Only oxybutinin is included in the BNF. This states that toxicity has been demonstrated in animal studies. Flavoxate is US category C, safety not established, use is only recommended if benefits (continence control) outweigh potential risks to fetus (Karch 1992)

Figure 11.2   *US drug categories adapted from Malseed et al. (1995)*

A No demonstrated fetal risk in humans during any stage of pregnancy

B No demonstrated risk in animal studies but no adequate studies in pregnant women

C Animal studies have shown adverse effects on the fetus but there are no adequate human studies

D Evidence of human fetal risk but the benefits from use of the drug may be acceptable despite the risks

X Animal or human studies have demonstrated fetal abnormalities, or adverse reaction reports give evidence of fetal risk (risk to a pregnant woman clearly outweighs possible benefits)

Figure 11.3   *Anticonvulsants in pregnancy*

Anticonvulsant therapy should be reviewed prior to conception, with a view to:

- Counselling: the risks of fits are greater than the risks of drugs. Sudden withdrawal of anticonvulsants may precipitate fits. Untreated, epilepsy tends to get worse. The risk of fetal abnormality is above that of the general population in people with untreated epilepsy. This may not be greatly increased by the use of monotherapy

- Gradual withdrawal and discontinuation if no fits have occurred for 5 years (Mackay & Evans 1995) or 4 years (Dichter 1991) or even less (Bloomfield 1996). This may take several months. All patients should be on the minimum effective doses possible

- Establishing monotherapy if at all possible

- Therapeutic monitoring and dose adjustment as necessary. If control of epilepsy has been poor before pregnancy, it is likely to worsen during pregnancy (Dichter 1991), due to hormonal changes

- Additional monitoring during pregnancy: alphafetoprotein and ultrasound

- Supplementation:
  – high-dose preconceptional folate
  – vitamin K in last trimester
  – vitamin D and calcium

Figure 11.4 *Multivitamins in pregnancy*

- Vitamin A is teratogenic in doses at and above 10 000 IU per day (Rothman *et al.* 1995). The threshold for fetal damage is only four times the RDA (Bloomfield 1996)
- Vitamin B_{12} is US category C. It is, however, an essential requirement
- Vitamin D is teratogenic in animals. Karch (1992) advises avoid doses above 400 IU per day. US category C
- Overdose of folic acid can precipitate convulsions in epileptics. US category A
- Menadiol (water-soluble vitamin K) is contraindicated in pregnancy Haemolytic anaemia of the newborn has occurred (BNF 1995) Phytomenadione is safe only in recommended doses for prophylaxis of haemorrhagic disease of the newborn. US category C

It is unwise to exceed the recommended RDA for other vitamins, such as niacin. Some substances marketed as 'vitamins' are toxic; for example vitamin B_{17} (laetrile) contains cyanide (Chetley 1995)

Raphael-Leff (1991) describes the psychological processes of pregnancy. These involve for all women some doubts about their ability to gestate and nourish a fetus. Such doubts may be worse where women live with an awareness that they have MS, and may feel themselves to be abnormal or defective. Women with a history of loss may under – or over – value the fetus. Undervaluing it is an insurance against the pain of further loss. To overvalue it is to invest in it the hopes which one does not invest in oneself. One major psychological task of pregnancy is to find a balance between identifying with the fetus, and thus laying the basis for the love the mother will feel for her child, and differentiating from it. Failure to differentiate can lead to psychological problems in the postnatal period, and such failure is more likely where the mother either over- or undervalues her fetus.

Midwives generally have little experience of disability and may overreact to perceived problems in care. There may be a tendency to overmedicalise, either because the nature of MS is misunderstood or to allay the helplessness staff may feel in the face of the uncontrollable. The pregnancy of a woman with MS is not high risk on account of the MS, although it may be for other reasons. Midwives and others may also disapprove of a woman with a disability having a child, or may feel the common embarrassment that disability evokes in the able bodied. Such feeling may lead to staff curtailing contact with the woman and thereby denying her information and choice. The message, for midwives, is clearly that the woman with MS is first and foremost a woman, second she is pregnant and planning on becoming a mother, and finally she has a condition that may require extra special care. Midwives should offer her continuity of carer, effective communication, choice in the decisions of childbirth and ultimately a feeling of control over the birth process whatever the medical condition.

A pregnant woman with MS is not necessarily at high risk and therefore needs and is entitled to the same level of information, leading to the same level of choice as any other woman. Care can be provided by a midwife who can take advice from other experts, such as obstetricians, neurologists and pharmacists, as necessary. The woman can be booked for a home birth, domino or hospital delivery. There may be a need for liaison with other health care professionals, for example physiotherapists, occupational therapists and incontinence nurses. Physiotherapists can advise about specific exercise plans to maximise mobility of affected limbs. Occupational therapists can advise about adaptations to either the woman's home or hospital wards. There may also be a need to liaise with an occupational therapist to assess the ergonomics of labour and postnatal wards, and recommend adaptations where necessary. Women with MS can be advised to exercise to their capacity, taking into account their individual mobility and the constraints of a growing pregnancy. Yoga classes take each woman's ability into account, and there is some anecdotal evidence that yoga ameliorates the symptoms of MS (ARMS 1993). If the woman's mobility is restricted, pelvic floor muscle exercises should be taught and advised to optimise the chance of a normal delivery (Campion 1990).

When a woman has chosen a hospital birth, visits to the labour and postnatal wards may be necessary to assess their accessibility and plan adaptations where necessary. This is particularly important if the woman has impaired vision; the more she can familiarise herself with the hospital during the antenatal period, the fewer problems she will have afterwards. If a woman uses a stick or wheelchair, it must be recognised that these aids are often experienced as an extension of her body. Sticks should never be moved away from her and chairs should never be leant on (Campion 1990). A woman in a wheelchair should never be moved without explanation or consent, except in dire emergency. If she is blind or visually impaired, antenatal group leaders should ensure that everyone introduces themselves. She should be given time to handle equipment, illustrations should be described, and she should be given written information that somebody else can read to her.

Women with MS should be given the same dietary advice as other pregnant women, with an emphasis on avoiding saturated fats and including fatty acids. Vegan or gluten-free diets may need to be examined by a nutritionist to check that they are adequate for pregnancy. It may be necessary to obtain a diary of what the woman has eaten for a number of typical days. Generally, when a woman has adopted such a diet, she is well informed about nutrition, often more so than health professionals.

The intrapartum period

There is little evidence available on the likely process and outcome of labour in women with MS. There is some anecdotal evidence that suggests that uncomplicated labours are more common. However, if a woman with MS is to have an uncomplicated labour, she must be given the opportunity to do so. Just as her pregnancy is not high risk on account of MS, neither is her labour, and an assumption of pathology is inappropriate. Each woman's capacity for active labour must be assessed individually, but the fact that a woman has MS does not mean that she needs to be confined to bed. The only form of analgesia that is contraindicated is spinal anaesthesia (Matthews *et al.* 1991), although the literature on the appropriateness of epidural anaesthesia is somewhat unclear. Campion (1990) states that anaesthetists may be reluctant to administer epidurals because the symptoms of certain complications, for example paralysis, tingling and numbness, are not easy to distinguish from the symptoms of MS. Matthews *et al.* (1991) make no mention of epidural anaesthesia in either the section on childbirth or that on surgery and anaesthetics.

Normal delivery is not contraindicated, although the MS Society in their literature consider that an assisted delivery may be necessary if muscle tone is poor. Certainly, MS is no indication for caesarean section, and there is some evidence to suggest that anaesthesia may precipitate a relapse (Matthews *et al.* 1991).

Similarly, MS alone is no indication for a hospital birth. It may be argued that women whose mobility or vision is compromised would be better off at home, where the surroundings are familiar and adapted to their needs, and the stresses of a new and unfamiliar environment are avoided. Infection rates are also lower at home (Campbell & Macfarlane 1994), and infection can be a cause of relapse or exacerbation of symptoms.

A recumbent or semirecumbent position throughout labour is not optimal for any woman, particularly not for a woman with MS, who may be vulnerable to pressure sores. There should not be an assumption that active birth is ruled out for a woman with MS. Alternative positions may be possible using furniture creatively. The woman may need actual physical support from the midwife and/or her partner. If she chooses to use a birthing pool or chair, these should be accessible or appropriately adapted.

The woman's partner is extremely important; he or she is likely to be familiar with her particular needs. But it is also important that midwives do not to fall into a 'Does she take sugar?' collusion with an able-bodied partner (Campion 1990).

Asepsis and prevention of infection are crucial, since infection and pyrexia can possibly induce relapses and certainly exacerbate symptoms.

The postnatal period

This is the time of increased risk of attack for women with MS, but there are measures that can be taken to minimise the risk.

The MS Society, in their unreferenced literature, state that bottlefeeding may be recommended if the woman is getting 'too tired' while breast-feeding. This advice is very misleading as artificial feeding involves the extra work of sterilisation and preparation. When a women breastfeeds her baby she sits or lies down and is able to rest for the duration of the feed. If the new mother has sufficient help, so that someone else could be feeding the baby, that help might be better used in caring for the mother and enabling her to breastfeed the baby. If the mother wants to breastfeed, and she is not taking any medication where breastfeeding is contraindi-cated, she should be offered all the support and encouragement necessary for her to do so. Breast milk is rich in essential fatty acids, and a mother with MS may want the reassurance that she is giving her baby, who is at a higher risk of developing MS than the general population, the best possible start. In addition, breastfed babies are generally healthier than bottlefed babies (Palmer 1988), and although while breastfeeding, a mother with MS may be increasing her chances of broken nights, she is reducing the risk of the stress of sickness in her baby. In addition, Smithers (1988) argues that for those mothers with MS with quite extensive physical prob-lems, the importance of breastfeeding (unless precluded by drug therapy) should be emphasised. It is something that only the mother could do for her child, and as such is of vital psychological importance.

Breastfeeding clearly offers both physiological and psychological advantages to the baby; in particular, breastfed babies suffer fewer gastrointestinal infections (Chetley 1995). Human studies on drug safety in breastfeeding are scarce. Some drugs are known to pass into breast milk and cause direct harm or drowsiness, which impairs breastfeeding (BNF 1995). The effects of drugs used in MS are outlined in Figure 11.5.

The postnatal period is one of psychological turbulence, which, like pregnancy, can be influenced by the woman's experience of MS. The diffi-dence and insecurity of a new mother may be worse if the MS has reduced her general confidence in herself. The midwife has an important role in helping the new mother believe in herself and believe in her ability to mother and nurture her new child.

Parenthood involves losses, including the loss of the lifestyle that existed before the child was born and, as in pregnancy, there is for the woman with MS the risk of past grief becoming an issue. The postnatal period is a time of increased risk of unhappiness, depression and psycho-logical disturbances for all women, and this is especially true for women with MS adjusting to the demands of motherhood.

Figure 11.5   *Breastfeeding and the drugs used in MS*

Diazepam	All benzodiazepines cause lethargy in the neonate. May impair feeding and weight gain
Baclofen	No consensus in the literature. Amount too small to be considered harmful (BNF 1995). Not recommended (Karch 1992)
Azathioprine	Immunosuppression is likely to be excessively hazardous. No information found in texts
Dantrolene	Contraindicated in breastfeeding (Karch 1992)
Corticosteroids	Corticosteroids are secreted in breast milk. Adrenal suppression in infant may lead to an Addisonian crisis if external steroids are abruptly withdrawn. Karch (1992) advises against breastfeeding
Anticonvulsants	These pass into breast milk. Barbiturates and ethosuximide are too sedating to be used during lactation. Manufacturers advise avoid phenytoin and newer anticonvulsants. Karch (1992) suggests that phenytoin is excessively hazardous. BNF (1995) states that phenytoin, valproate and carbamazepine are given in quantities too small to be harmful. However, hypersensitivity responses to carbamazepine have occurred in infants, making breastfeeding hazardous (Karch 1992)
Multivitamins	Intake should be in line with recommended daily allowances. Some vitamins – vitamin A, vitamin D and menadione – are potentially toxic

The new baby may evoke complex feelings. If it is physically well, there may be tremendous pride and relief, but there may also be feelings that the baby is absolutely perfect, combined with envy that the baby is whole. If the baby is not well, the guilt may be complicated by doubts surrounding the right to have a child in the first place.

Women with MS may be particularly vulnerable to postnatal depression, which may be because the woman may feel herself to be deficient or inadequate. This may be associated with previous feelings towards the baby: as a fetus the child may have been overvalued, but once it is born, the loss and sense of depletion may be overwhelming. If the baby was previously undervalued, the guilt may be overpowering. In any case, the healthy baby's potential for life and growth can be painful to contemplate when the woman's own potential at best is doubtful and at worst severely limited.

For women with MS, common responses to the stresses and strains of parenthood may be met with fear and alarm. For example, it is not unusual for new mothers to be forgetful, have difficulty in concentrating and find themselves preoccupied with their new baby, but for women with MS these symptoms have sinister connections. Women with MS may be confused and fearful of what are essentially normal aspects of the puerperium and the early days of motherhood. The symptoms described do not necessarily mean that the condition is deteriorating but are frequently a normal part of the transition to motherhood.

Some contraceptives may be contraindicated for women with MS. Oral contraception has no deleterious effect on MS, but if the woman's mobility is impaired, it may be inadvisable because of the increased risk of deep vein thrombosis and pulmonary embolus. An intrauterine device may be contraindicated if sensation is impaired, as symptoms of pelvic inflammatory disease might be missed. As previously, the woman should be encouraged to seek the advice of an expert in family planning, who should take a holistic view of the woman's needs.

The midwife may need to help the family in assessing how to reduce fatigue as much as possible. The family may need to consider what help is available and how it can be mobilised. Together they might consider what has worked for the woman in the past to prevent relapses and has helped to reduce the severity of symptoms. The midwife might advise the parents to adopt a contingency plan to deal with any problems that might arise with the care of their baby if the mother were to have a relapse of her illness.

The woman should be warned of the possibility of excessive breast fullness and the temporary rise in temperature that can result, and be advised to take paracetamol.

OTHER SOURCES OF HELP AND ADVICE

If the woman does have problems in handling the baby, there is a residential facility at Mary Marlborough Lodge in Oxford where mothers and babies are assessed with regard to needs and possibilities in terms of practical help with lifting and handling. They accept referrals nationwide. Women are usually referred by doctors, but can be referred by a social worker if the local authority will agree to the funding. Women may also refer themselves if they pay privately. Staff at the Lodge will also assess pregnant women and their partners, preferably during the second or third trimester. Midwives can make referrals provided they have ascertained that funding is available.

The MS Society runs an Advice Line and has offices in London, Edinburgh and Belfast. The Multiple Sclerosis Resource Centre (formerly ARMS – Action for Research into Multiple Sclerosis) offers individualised support and assessment, particularly with reference to physiotherapy, nutrition and counselling. The MS Unit at the Central Middlesex Hospital in London will take referrals from outside the district if they are accompanied by funding.

CONCLUSIONS

It is difficult to say how a midwife might need to adapt her practice to accommodate a woman with MS, since it is impossible to know in advance what those needs are. Women with MS do have special needs, and because those needs are entirely idiosyncratic they demand an individual and special woman-centred approach.

Campion (1990) describes some attitudes that childbearing women with disabilities often encounter, which can be more distressing than the disability itself. She offers advice to health care professionals, including midwives, saying that midwives should remember that the environment familiar to midwives is alien and frightening for pregnant clients. She warns midwives to make allowances for couples who appear defensive, as they often feel they are being scrutinised and judged as potential parents. She reminds midwives of the importance of working as part of a team and at the same time recognising the expertise of the woman in the management of her disability. Effective communication is, as always, the key to effective care.

MS is of relevance to midwives because it is relevant to childbearing women. It offers a challenge to midwifery practice in subtle and indirect ways. A woman with MS may be indistinguishable from a fit and healthy woman as far as the midwife is concerned, and will therefore have no special needs, or she may be considerably handicapped and require flexibility from the midwife both in the ingenuity needed to adapt the hospital environment and in her attitude. A midwife needs to keep an open mind on hearing that a woman has MS, regard her as the expert on her own condition and draw up with her an individualised care plan, not just for the birth but also for the antenatal and postnatal periods.

REFLECTIONS

A woman with MS, in common with other people with a disability, presents a challenge to the basic assumptions and attitudes of the able bodied. However, the greatest challenge such a woman will pose is the opportunity that arises to deal with the issues of mortality, fear of illness and vulnerability. A man with muscular dystrophy once wrote, 'for the able bodied world we are a representation of many of the things they most fear, tragedy, loss, dark and the unknown. Involuntary we walk, or more often sit, in the valley of the shadow of death. Contact with us throws up in people's faces the fact of sickness and death in the world' (Hunt 1982).

To some extent midwives are used to dealing with these issues, since birth intimately evokes the possibility of death. Menzies-Lyth (1988) states:

> It seems that a sizeable component of [the maternal] role concerned death and mourning. The baby may perhaps be regarded as the reminder of mortality, even if not an ugly one. Birth is a reminder of death if only because, in a sense, it is the opposite, the final establishment of a new life. Birth is frequently experienced as a moment of great danger for both mother and child, for which strenuous survival preparations are made. In the ensuing period the realistic facility of the baby, its vulnerability, its lack of capacity for unassisted survival, add to the feeling of hazard. Not is it only a matter of physical survival. The situation is equally fraught on the psychological side. The baby has no more capacity for unassisted survival and effective development psychologically than physically.

Just as the mother assists the physical and psychological survival of her baby, so a midwife does this for the clients in her care. Mothers and midwives normally do this unconsciously, but some clients cause psychological turbulence for midwives. Among these might well be women with MS. If midwives can remain open to their clients' needs and wishes without retreating unduly to counterproductive psychological defences, they will have met and overcome the greatest challenge.

ACKNOWLEDGEMENTS

The author of this chapter would like to acknowledge the advice, comments and helpful suggestions made by Dr Rosie Jones, Linda K Brown, Dr Sue Jordan and Sheila Hunt.

REFERENCES

Action for Research into Multiple Sclerosis (ARMS) 1993 *A Demographic Profile*. Uxbridge: ARMS

Bloomfield T 1996 Principles of prescribing in pregnancy. *Prescriber* 19 Jan: 66–70

British National Formulary (BNF) 1995 No 3. London: BMA and the Royal Pharmaceutical Society of Great Britain

British Society of Rehabilitation Medicine (BSRM) 1993 *Multiple Sclerosis: A working party report of the British Society of Rehabilitation Medicine*. London: BSRM

Campbell R, Macfarlane A 1994 *Where to be Born? The Debate and the Evidence*, 2nd edn. Oxford: National Perinatal Epidemiology Unit

Campion M Jain 1990 *The Baby Challenge*. London: Routledge

Chetley A 1995 *Problem Drugs*. London: Zed Books.

Dichter M 1991 The epilepsies and convulsive disorders. In Wilson J, Braunwald E, Isseleacher K *et al.* (eds) *Harrison's Principles and Practice of Medicine.* New York: McGraw Hill

Forti A, Segal J (undated) *MS and Pregnancy.* London: ARMS

Hunt P 1982 Cited in ARMS 1993 *Talking about MS.* Uxbridge: ARMS

Karch A 1992 *Handbook of Drugs and Nursing Process,* 2nd edn. Philadelphia: JB Lippincott

MacKay H, Evans T 1995 Gynaecology and obstetrics. In Tierney LM, McPhee SJ, Papadakis M (eds) *Current Medical Diagnosis and Treatment.* Norwalk, CT: Lange Medical

Malseed RT, Goldstein FJ, Balkon N 1995 *Pharmacology: Drug therapy and nursing considerations,* 4th edn. Philadelphia: JB Lippincott

Matthews B 1985 *Multiple Sclerosis: the facts.* Oxford: Oxford University Press

Matthews WB, Compston A, Allen I, Martin C 1991 *MacAlpine's Multiple Sclerosis.* London: Churchill Livingstone

Medawar C 1992 *Power and Dependence: Social audit on the safety of medicines.* London: Social Audit

Menzies-Lyth I 1988 *Containing Anxiety in Institutions.* London: Free Association Books

Palmer G 1988 *The Politics of Breast Feeding.* London: Pandora Press

Raphael-Leff J 1991 *Psychological Processes of Childbearing.* London: Chapman & Hall.

Rothman K, Moore L, Singer M, Nguyen U, Mannino S, Milunsky A 1995 Teratogenicity of high vitamin A intake. *New England Journal of Medicine* **333**(21):1369–73

Smithers K 1988 Practical problems of mothers who have multiple sclerosis. *Midwife, Health Visitor and Community Nurse* **24** (5):167–8

USEFUL ADDRESSES.

Mary Marlborough Disability Centre
Nuffield Orthopaedic Centre NHS Trust
Windmill Road
Oxford OX3 7LD   Tel: (01865) 741155

Multiple Sclerosis Society of Great Britain and Northern Ireland
25 Effie Road
London SW6 1EL   (Help line) 0171–610 7171

MS Society in Scotland
2A North Charlotte Street
Edinburgh EH2 4HR   Tel: 0131–225 3600

MS Society Northern Ireland Office
34 Annadale Avenue
Belfast BT7 3JJ   Tel: (01232) 644914

MS Unit (formerly part of ARMS)
Central Middlesex Hospital
Acton Lane
London NW10 7NS   Tel: 0181-453 2332/2337

Multiple Sclerosis Resource Centre
4a Chapel Hill
Stansted
Essex CM24 8AG   Tel: 01279 817101

National Childbirth Trust: ParentAbility
Alexandra House
Oldham Terrace
Acton
London W3 6NH   Tel: 0181-992 8637

RADAR (Royal Association for Disability and Rehabilitation)
25 Mortimer Street
London W1N 8AB   Tel: 0171-250 3222

SPOD (Sexual and Personal Relationships of the Disabled)
286 Camden Road
London N7 OBJ   Tel: 0171-607 8851

Yoga for Health Foundation
Ickwell Bury
Northill
Biggleswade
Bedfordshire SG18 9BS   Tel: (01767) 627271

CHAPTER TWELVE

The challenge of change in the organisation of midwifery care

Sheila C. Hunt

The aim of this chapter is to help midwives understand, analyse and face changes in the organisation, philosophy and practice of midwifery. The chapter will be divided into two key sections: the analysis of change and the management of change. The analysis section will consider the origins and pressures for change and explore the key change management theories.

The second section will discuss aspects of managing change and consider why individuals and organisations resist change. This section is not for 'managers only' but for all midwives who manage the care of women and their partners, or are themselves managed by professional and other managers. Options in selecting strategies for change will be debated, as will some of the apparently easy answers offered by 'management gurus' and theorists. The final section offers a summary and conclusion.

THE ANALYSIS OF CHANGE

Why does childbirth have to change?

Over many years, midwives have become increasingly aware of the need to keep themselves up to date and be well informed. The explosion in midwifery literature is evidence of the growing complexity and detail associated with what has until recently been a practical skill passed on from one generation to another with the help of a single text book affectionately referred to as 'Maggie Myles'. In this book, 'Challenges in Midwifery Care', each of the chapters has explored aspects of midwifery practice that present those who care with a challenge. Some of the conditions described will be part of the day-to-day practice of midwifery for some midwives, while other conditions are so rare that they will only be encountered by a few. But there is now a new and additional challenge facing midwives: childbirth has to change, and the way in which care is organised must also change. Maternity care must be 'women centred, concentrating on meeting the needs of the women for whom the service is intended' (Department of Health 1993, p 5).

165

Most midwives will meet poverty, deprivation, illness, disease and sadness in their professional practice, but as we approach the next millennium there is no doubt that all midwives will have to come face to face with the uncertainty, the fear and the challenge of change. Midwives are well equipped to give special care to the special people described in this book, but many will now be seeking someone to understand and care for them, as carers, as they face a period of unprecedented change in the way in which they practise midwifery.

The origins and pressures for change

The policy background to such a major change has been well described by Sandall (1995), who records the impact of government reports, the efforts of consumer groups and pressure groups, as well as the desire of the government to emphasise the so-called 'voice of the consumer' while challenging unacceptable professional power. Sandall describes the new work of midwives as being required to demonstrate post-Fordist flexibility, while Wilson (1992) describes the new 'enterprise culture' as the driving force behind many of the current changes. The Conservative government of the past decade and a half, with the emergence of Thatcherism, is probably the main force for change in all public sector activities. Fordism (*c.*1930–70) describes the long period of economic growth associated with the type of industrial and economic organisation of the time. For example, organisations were set up to mass produce single products, such as Ford motor cars, technologies focused on single products, semiskilled work forces were represented by large trade unions, and change was seen as a natural process of facilitating even more mass production and consumption of goods.

Post-Fordism, on the other hand, encourages organisations to specialise, produce goods for niche markets, increase competitiveness, decentralise, down-size, adopt lean structures, subcontract, employ multiskilled workers alongside part-time, contracted and temporary workers, probably most importantly recognise the value of the consumer in 'driving up' quality, and finally develop organisational cultures that produce employers who are fanatical followers of the company aim (Atkinson 1984). Charles Handy, in 'The Age of Unreason' (1991), describes his vision of a post-Fordist society in which there are new rules and a constant requirement for change in attitudes and working practices. He could have been writing for midwives in the last decade of the twentieth century. Listening to what customers want and then meeting those needs efficiently and effectively is the message from major international corporations, as well as from providers of public sector services (Drucker 1990; Wille 1992). Midwifery is not immune from these pressures; it operates in a society in which the key message appears to be 'Know your rights and demand your choice'. Virginia Bottomley as Secretary of State for Health, offered a message at the start of 'Changing Childbirth' (Department of Health 1993). She said:

> At the heart of the NHS reforms is the need for health authorities to listen more and more to what users feel about the health service they require. The thinking in the group's [Expert Maternity Group] report is totally in keeping with that philosophy.

In each of the four countries of the UK, considerable attention has been directed towards the provision and organisation of maternity care. In Scotland, a policy review was undertaken in 1993, with subsequent recommendations set out in the document 'Provision of Maternity Services in Scotland: A policy review'. In Northern Ireland, a Maternity Unit Study Group's report was accepted by the Department of Health and Social Services and the document 'Delivering Choice: Report of the Northern Ireland Maternity Unit Study Group' was subsequently published in 1994. In Wales, the 'Protocol for Investment in Health Gain for Maternal and Early Child Health' highlighted the importance of providing childbearing women with greater choice, control and continuity of carer. In England, 'Changing Childbirth' was published in August 1993, and changes in the maternity services have become inevitable.

'Changing Childbirth' (p 14) reported that, for many women, continuity of carer was one of the most important aspects of their care. Women felt that meeting the same midwife improved communication between the woman, her partner and the midwife. Oakley *et al.* (1990) provided evidence of the benefits of social support in pregnancy where the woman had the support of a known carer. Hodnett (1993) demonstrated that women who know their carer feel more supported and subsequently feel more in control of their birth experience. Green *et al.* (1990) demonstrate that, even when things go wrong, women are more likely to feel satisfied about their birth experience if they feel in control and involved in the decision-making processes.

So improving continuity of carer improves communication between midwives and the women they care for. A partnership is then more likely to develop in which the woman has greater awareness and understanding of the choices open to her and is able to appreciate the responsibilities associated with her choices. The key to improving women's satisfaction with their birth experience would appear to be organising care so as to provide continuity of carer. This reorganisation is happening in maternity units and community areas all over the UK. Midwives who for many years have worked in the antenatal clinic or in the labour ward, or on night duty, or as community midwives, who have little to do with intrapartum care, are being asked, cajoled or forced to change the ways in which they work.

Other pressures for change

An analysis of the external forces of change in the organisation of the maternity services is relatively straightforward. The major impetus for change comes from government policy, but other factors are also important. Technological changes are continuous and a major pressure for change. Developments in the treatment of infertility, congenital disorders, fetal surgery, ultrasound, prenatal testing and neonatal care technology all have an effect on the demand and supply of maternity services. Demographic changes, especially in relation to the numbers and ages of childbearing women in an area, alter demand for care, as do geographical issues such as where people live, where they want to give birth and how they travel. Major international events can produce pressure for change although not directly affecting the maternity services; for example, the earthquake in Kobe in Japan led to an acute shortage of computer memory. Computers are an essential part of all technological developments, so even earthquakes in remote countries have an effect on midwifery care. The collapse of the Berlin Wall opened new trading opportunities for many companies, including those selling baby milks and fetal monitoring equipment. New demand leads to economic growth and further technological developments. Finally, there are changes in the law of the country as new case law is established. It is not unreasonable to think that the first successful civil law case suing an obstetrician for an unnecessary caesarean section might change the practice of obstetrics. The world of maternity care may only appear to feel ripples from external events, but public sector organisations such as health care and education are as vulnerable as are large multinational companies. In many large companies, the major triggers for change from outside the organisation are falling profits, increased competition, changing consumer demands, loss of market share and other financial disasters. The economic health of the public sector depends to a large extent on the wealth created by business and industry (Drucker 1990).

Change also comes from inside organisations. Ideas change, policies change and, according to Kotter and Hesketh (1992), major cultural change within large organisations is often created by the appointment of new Chief Executives. They refer to British Airways (Lord King and Sir Colin Marshall), British Leyland (Sir Michael Edwards and Sir Graham Day), General Electric (Jack Welch) and ICI (Sir John Harvey-Jones). Many midwives will recognise the feeling of a 'new broom sweeping clean'.

For some midwives, the job itself changes. Perhaps an elderly friendly GP retires from their patch or the Senior Midwife moves on. Hospitals close, reorganisations happen and change becomes a familiar part of everyday life.

It is very important for midwives to spend time thinking and analysing the change that is around them. It is easy to slip into a belief that today's problems have one simple cause: the government's NHS reforms, but this is far too simplistic and ignores the many external forces that bring about change. Change is not peculiar to this decade, although its pace has certainly accelerated; it was in the fourth century BC that Pliny the Elder was reported to have said, 'The only certainty is that nothing is certain'.

THEORIES AND MODELS OF CHANGE

The most famous process model of change was described by Lewin in 1951. Most subsequent models are variations on this and consist of a series of stages over a period of time. Lewin saw change as passing through three distinct phases: unfreezing, change and refreezing. He argued that any organisation, individual or group that was to change had to be unfrozen or freed from their previous stable and comfortable state, then changed and then refrozen. His assumption was that once a change had happened and been accepted, that would be the end of the matter and no further change would be required of the refrozen organisation. Perhaps that was the case in 1951.

Marris (1986) compares and contrasts change and bereavement. He argues that both loss and change disrupt our ability to find meaning in experience, and it is in periods of recovery that individuals attempt to give meaning to the present. There are many midwives who, when faced with a reorganised maternity service, feel the same symptoms of grief – grief for the loss of the old way of doing things and a great reluctance to accept change. Kubler-Ross (1984), in her seminal work on death, described periods of shock, denial, anger, bargaining, depression and later acceptance. These are not dissimilar to the emotions felt by many as change is forced upon them. Marris argues that rituals and ceremonies can help individuals to adapt to change, as can the support of colleagues who share the experience. He believes that people need time to let go or unfreeze and need time to talk about the loss. He emphasises the importance of valuing the past and not falling into the trap that the new is bound to be better. Mead and Bryar (1992) have also used a theoretical framework of loss and attachment to analyse the changes involved in introducing the nursing process and primary nursing.

In the late 1980s and early 1990s, simple process models to explain and understand change were being rejected. Isabella (1990) argued that the culture and complexity of the organisation have to be understood and interpreted and that, even within organisations, change does not always follow the same pattern. Isabella studied 40 managers from medium-sized financial companies, all of which were undergoing substantial changes. From her interview data, she established four key stages of interpretation.

These stages can be compared with those described by Lewin as unfreezing, change and refreezing. The stages are anticipation, confirmation, culmination and aftermath. This is quite a useful model and can be used to explain and understand changes in a maternity hospital.

Anticipation

This is the stage at which rumours abound; some midwives have read the journals, some midwives on courses have heard about 'Changing Childbirth', there is talk of a new manager or a change agent. Each midwife constructs her version of reality; she telephones other midwives, and together they try to connect pieces of the puzzle. Some eagerly anticipate the change, some begin to make other plans.

Confirmation

Anticipation is confirmed, but there is little objective reality. There is information and misinformation, and frames of reference are based on previous experience. Each midwife has her own idea of how things may develop.

Culmination

At this stage, individuals amend their prior interpretation of forthcoming events. With more information, individuals look for clues from which to derive new meanings. Some midwives will read more, attend meetings, ask more questions.

Aftermath

This is the final stage during which the events or the new team, or the new rotas, or the new case loads are tested and tried. Reality is confirmed, and the winners and losers easily identified. Isabella argued that this is when the effects of change of the whole are interpreted by individuals and the question is asked, 'So what does this mean for me?' Individual midwives will make predictions and decide whether or not to see the change through or look for alternatives inside or outside the organisation. Change, Isabella argues, is not just a sequence but a process fuelled by a variety of interpretations, each of which provides a spur to action, creates the vision and sustains the energies of those caught up in the change (Wilson 1992, p 83).

Lancaster and Lancaster (1982) offer an interesting model to assist in understanding individual and group responses to change. The change may be seen by some as a challenge and by others as a threat. Table 12.1 sets out Rogers' thinking and describes how different individuals or groups within groups may be divided.

Table 12.1   *Responses to change*

Category	Percentage
The innovators: enthusiastic and venturesome	2
The early adopters: respectful and obedient	13
The early majority: deliberate and thoughtful	34
The late majority: sceptical and suspicious	35
The laggards: traditional and reluctant to change	16
The saboteurs: dangerous, devious and hidden	Unknown??

(modified from Rogers 1962 and Lancaster and Lancaster 1982)

Rogers argues that, in any group, 2 per cent will be leaders or innovators of change. This small group, or even one individual, will lead the change. Innovators are usually very enthusiastic, energetic and keen to make change happen as soon as possible. They are often, but not always, the formal leaders. They see the vision, have a clear view of how things should be and rarely lose sight of that vision. They can be sent away to gather more information but will always return to continue their mission. They are persuasive, determined and active.

The group Rogers refers to as 'early adopters' make up 13% of the total. They are usually quick to come on board and become the friends and disciples of the innovators. The 'innovators' and 'early adopters', joined by the 'early majority', provide a powerful force for change. The 'late majority', around 35 per cent, remain sceptical and need much more information before they will move with the early majority. They listen to all sides but take note of what the remaining 16 per cent (the laggards) are saying. The 'laggards' hold back and are very resistant to change.

What Rogers' model does not include is a very active group well known in midwifery circles called 'the saboteurs'. This group, which can be great in number, are very difficult to discover and manage. Frequently, they are secretive about their views and appear to be contained within the late majority. Sometimes they appear to be part of the early majority and find their way on to task groups and planning teams. Their mission is to undermine, sabotage and prevent the team moving forward. They often present logical, well-prepared arguments and can seem plausible, but their mission is simply to prevent change from happening. Unfortunately, the empirical evidence suggests that they secretly undermine the activities of those committed to change and, by stealth, deception and the spreading of half truths and untruths, are able to sabotage the best of schemes.

This is a useful model that helps those involved in planning change to be aware of the dynamics of many groups. Saboteurs are not always present, but if the progress towards change is especially slow, it may be worth considering whether there is a saboteur on the team. Phillips (1983) has also produced a simple model, based on Lewin's work, which is helpful in seeing the process of change as a series of discrete changes over time. The model assumes that 'top management' has diagnosed the need for change. (Using a familiar analogy, this 'top down' initiative can be described as the 'shower approach' as opposed to the 'bidet' or 'bottom up' approach, in which the initiative and drive come from those closely involved in the change.)

Figure 12.1, based on Phillips (1983), describes the phases in the organisation of change.

Figure 12.1   *Stages in the organisation of change*

───────────────▶ Acceleration of momentum ─────────────────▶

STAGE 1 Creating a sense of concern	STAGE 2 Developing a specific commitment to change	STAGE 3 Pushing for major change	STAGE 4 Reinforcing and consolidating the new vision
First serious concern	First effort to change	Real commitment to action	Evidence of turn around
		First results	Full results of change

Phillip's model depends on key individuals in the organisation being active in stage 3. The managers or leaders must motivate all others to bring about the change. Phillips argues that managers must pull, in unison and in the same direction, the same 'change levers'. The change levers are traditionally described in 'Leavitt's Diamond' (1964) (Figure 12.2).

Figure 12.2   *Leavitt's Diamond (adapted from Leavitt 1964)*

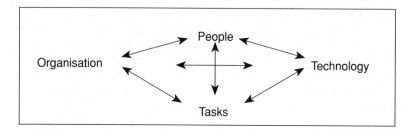

According to Kirkbridge (1993), managers can intervene in the four key areas of 'people', 'the organisation', 'technology' and 'tasks' to bring about change.

In midwifery, one of the key areas in which managers might need to intervene is 'people'; perhaps a midwife has only worked in the antenatal clinic since qualifying and needs more delivery suite experience; here staff can be prepared for their new roles through continuing education and by the support of a supervisor of midwives. The manager may need to act by increasing staff in community areas and reducing staff on underused antenatal wards. In Leavitt's Diamond, it is important to note that each of the four areas is connected and pressure on one lever produces corresponding pressure in other areas. For example, the introduction of a new information system in a maternity unit will affect people, the tasks they do and the organisation itself. In Phillips' model, the final stage of 'reinforcing and consolidating the new vision' aims at creating the capacity for further change and a willingness to adapt to subsequent change more quickly.

Most of the models described assume the existence of a process. Plant (1987) has proposed a need, commitment and shared vision model aimed at helping managers to steer the organisation through change and the consequential trauma to the workforce. However, many managers and academics are beginning to reject these and other simplistic models and see them as of use only in explaining what is happening rather than in how to help to make it happen. Most of the literature focuses on theories of change rather than on theories of changing. As such, it tends to be suitable for observers of change rather than practitioners of change. The process of change is complex and exceedingly difficult to achieve. The nature of the human animal is to cling to that which is familiar, and, for reasons as basic as ensuring survival, attempts are made to resist change. The new buzz word in understanding change is 'culture'. The key to bringing about change, according to Ouchi (1981), Deal and Kennedy (1982), Peters and Waterman (1982), Atkinson (1990), Brown (1992) and many others, is to analyse, understand and then try to change the culture. This will be discussed in the next section.

MANAGING CHANGE

Analysing and understanding resistance to change

Managing change is mainly about understanding and dealing with resistance. The most common response to a change proposal is a series of angry objections, some carefully considered logical objections and some ill-considered, illogical objections often unrelated to the proposed change.

According to Basil and Cook (1974) the origins of change can be analysed and diagnosed in three major classifications: structural–institutional, technological and social–behavioural. They argue that change is impacting on all facets of society, creating new dimensions and great uncertainty, and that the key issue facing managers today is how to manage change. In practice, this means that managers are dealing with new government and European regulations and directives, new services and demands, technological developments and a rapidly changing workforce. Individuals and organisations have to develop strategies and structures to manage change effectively, but at the root of many difficulties lies the ability of individuals and organisations to resist change. Kotter and Schlesinger (1988) say that managers need to be aware of the four most common reasons for people resisting change. These are a desire not to lose something of value, a misunderstanding of the change and its implications, a belief that the change does not make sense for the organisation and a low tolerance for change.

Harvey-Jones (1989, p 147) says of change:

> the processes (of change) are almost certainly disruptive and require adaptation to an astounding degree, adaptation which ultimately can be made on an individual and personal level

while Nadler and Tushman (1989, p 198) state:

> one of the greatest strengths of organisations is that they contain tremendous forces for stability. They are able to withstand threats and challenges to the established order. The flip side of this characteristic is that organisations (and particularly successful ones) can be inherently resistant to change, particularly change that undermines strongly held values and beliefs.

For many midwives facing the challenge of the changes set out in 'Changing Childbirth', their well-established, cherished beliefs about how midwifery care ought to be given are being challenged. They argue at conferences and study days that there was little wrong with the old familiar ways and that few women ever complained. Their fundamental beliefs and values are being challenged, and a great deal of energy is being put into resistance. Many believe that something of value may be lost (for example, continuity of carer for women whose pregnancies are considered high risk), some misunderstand the change and feel it is a cost-cutting exercise, some believe that midwifery does not need reorganising and is fine as it is, and many feel that their capacity for change is now exhausted as a result of the health service reorganisation.

In psychological terms, the pain and uncertainty of resistance can create dissonance. This is the force or energy that can motivate an individual to take action to alleviate the discomfort caused, in this case, by the mismatch between the way things are and the way the maternity services are going to be. Resistance is the force exerted to prevent change; it can be individual and/or organisational, it can be active or passive and as a force it has to be understood and managed.

Leigh (1988) defines resistance as 'any conduct that tries to maintain the status quo in the face of pressure to change it'. It is accepted that the human animal prefers the familiar and is more comfortable with the aspects of his or her life that have been learnt through habit. Individuals faced with change, especially on the scale proposed in the maternity services, experience a range of emotions, the most common of which is fear. Harvey-Jones (1989) says that fear is an intensely personal matter and that no two individuals' fears are the same; as such, fear cannot be dealt with in generalised terms. Fear and uncertainty create mistrust and more fear. There may be role confusion and apprehension, threats to self-esteem, and anxiety about income and the ability to cope with new demands, with responses ranging from active, open, hostile, aggressive behaviour to passive resistance, characterised by regressive behaviour, non-learning and protests. Active resistance may take many forms, including slowing down, personal withdrawal (taking extended sick leave), committing minor errors, working to rule or to the letter of the UKCC Rules, or even deliberate sabotage. Those who resist may simply be afraid.

Not all change is resisted – where there are suitable rewards change may be welcomed – but resistance is bound to be a feature when midwives see themselves being asked to take on greater responsibility and work longer hours on more flexible rotas, for the same or less financial reward. Salary increases and improved status are likely to be accepted and to be used more frequently to motivate reluctant midwives. There is little evidence that improved status and greater autonomy are sufficient in themselves to overcome resistance to change.

According to Leigh (1988) and others, change can be resisted for many reasons, including: fear of loss; insecurity and fear of promotion; a memory of a previous badly handled change; a misunderstanding of change and its implications; insufficient information and no perceived benefits; a belief that changes are wrong for the organisation; uncertainty in relation to freedom and constraints; inexperience in implementing change; existing psychological and social commitments to current products or services, processes and organisations; complacency; powerful trade union attitudes to change; the complexity and fear of uncertainty; and a belief that if management want it, it must be wrong!

Finally, it is important to acknowledge that there may be legitimate resistance to change. It is very important to listen carefully to those who object to change. It is easy to label individuals as laggards or hostile resisters when it is more important to listen to their concerns, however trivial they may first appear. It is reasonable for those planning change to anticipate opposition, but it is unreasonable to assume that all opposition is irrational.

Overcoming resistance

Harvey-Jones (1989), perhaps optimistically, states that it is better by far to achieve some change that may self-accelerate than to expend all the available energy on resistance. He advocated careful planning and selection of appropriate strategies. He anticipated that although he could change his Board (at ICI) in the first year, it would take some 4 or 5 years to begin to change attitudes and people. Perhaps, like Machiavelli (1513) and many midwifery managers in the 1990s, he has considered that:

> There is nothing more difficult to carry out nor more doubtful of success nor more dangerous to handle, than to initiate a new order of things.

Most writers agree that there are no quick-fix answers to overcoming resistance, although, as Johnson and Scholes (1989) argue, it is unrealistic to suppose that change can be implemented if current beliefs and assumptions remain the same. Overcoming resistance to change involves understanding organisations and how change takes place as well as understanding how individuals in that organisation think, believe and act.

Change and culture

Lorsch (1986) recommends a culture audit as a method of increasing understanding of the organisation and its values. The audit would help to define beliefs about goals, about distinctive competencies and the product or service on offer, and about the relationship between managers and employees. For many midwives, the chance to attempt to define their own philosophy of midwifery, as suggested by Bryar (1995), would be an important first stage in defining the culture of their organisation. The challenge to managers would be to respect and value the existing culture while encouraging flexibility and free thinking. Change has to be planned after careful analysis of the particular environment; while some general principles can be established, it is unlikely that a standard format will suit every maternity unit.

It appears that resistance can be overcome, at least in part, by careful diagnosis and understanding of the culture. This analysis, together with specific training and education programmes, is an important part of the preliminary work of change. Sometimes individuals, structures and systems and aspects of the interpersonal culture all have to be changed prior to the planned change (Goodstein & Burke 1992).

Schein (1986) believes that, in managing any change, the employee has to become motivated to unlearn something and then replace it with new learning. It is suggested that this is best achieved by identifying with a new role model or by finding information most relevant to the problem. The change, according to Schein, is then thought of as cognitive restructuring or redefinition, resulting in new perceptions, new feelings, new judgements and ultimately new behaviours. At this stage, dissonance is no longer a feature and resistance has subsided. Schein describes the role of the manager as a 'change agent' who may act and intervene at any of Lewin's stages. Schein also emphasises that unfreezing is a lengthy process and change frequently fails because this phase is too short or too ill considered.

Unlearning and relearning both require a culture change and need cultural leadership to make it happen. Leaders help to define culture and to create an environment in which change and innovation are the norm. Kanter (1983) found that segmentalist, low-innovating companies share 10 qualities (Figure 12.3). These qualities stifle innovation and are a common feature of the intensely hierarchical NHS, which has traditionally placed more emphasis on seniority than ability. In changing the organisation and philosophy of midwifery care, some of the traditional ways of the NHS, which are deeply entrenched in the culture, will need to be unlearnt.

All organisations, departments and even wards have a culture. It may not be the one that they want nor the one best suited to taking on a major change. Kanter (1983) believes that the skill of leaders lies in their ability to see the new way and then translate that vision into more concrete terms. She also believes that success breeds success, and where there is a culture of pride based on achievement, people's confidence in themselves and others increases. They become braver, achieve more and work better in teams. One of the tasks ahead is that of creating a culture in maternity units in which new ideas are welcomed, and midwives are trusted, supported and frequently praised. Midwives should be able to give care in units and homes where mistakes that are not dangerous or life-threatening are tolerated and used constructively as part of peer review and reflective learning; midwives need to be able to work where they feel empowered to take decisions about care without fear of personal criticism and attack. There are longstanding traditions and attitudes in nursing and midwifery that are, as part of the culture, passed from one generation to the next and as such are very difficult to change. Sometimes, when change seems impossible, outside consultants can be brought in to analyse and diagnose the difficulties. They study the culture and, as outsiders, are often able to see clearly what is hidden from those who are familiar with the setting. They produce a report that sets out those aspects which are preventing change and preventing improvements in care for women and their families. The words of an external consultant, written in a glossy brochure, for which vast sums of money have often been paid, are frequently the catalyst for change. New appointments from outside the NHS Trust or area have a similar function. It seems that when an outsider tells an organisation those things that they often already know, the 'unfreezing' and changing can begin.

Figure 12.3   *Rules for stifling innovation (taken from RM Kanter,* The Change Masters: Corporate Entrepreneurs at Work, *1983. London, Routledge, p. 101. Reproduced by permission.)*

Rules for stifling innovation

1. Regard any new idea from below with suspicion – because it's new and it's from below.

2. Insist that people who need your approval to act go through several other levels of management to get their signatures.

3. Ask departments or individuals to challenge and criticise each other's proposals. (That saves you the job of deciding, you just pick the survivors.)

4. Express your criticisms freely, and withhold praise. This keeps people on their toes. Let people know that they can be fired at any time.

5. Treat identification of problems as signs of failure, to discourage people from letting you know when something in their area is not working.

6. Control everything carefully. Make sure people count everything that can be counted very carefully, frequently.

7. Make decisions to reorganise or change policies in secret and spring them on people unexpectedly. That also keeps them on their toes.

8. Make sure that requests for information are fully justified, and make sure that it is not given out to managers freely. (You don't want data in the wrong hands.)

9. Assign to lower levels of management, in the name of delegation and participation, responsibility for figuring out how to cut back, lay off, move people around or otherwise implement threatening decisions you have made. And get them to do it quickly.

10. Above all else, never forget that you, the higher ups, already know everything that is important about this business.

Force field analysis

Management texts are awash with frameworks, recipes, checklists and training games designed to help managers to analyse change, predict the consequences of failure, handle resistance and move from the actual to the optimal. All are useful in promoting thought and preventing the overenthusiastic innovator from rushing into failure.

Lewin (1951), whose model of unfreezing, changing and refreezing has been discussed above, argued that organisations exist in a state of equilibrium or *status quo* that is not conducive to change. This state of equilibrium is a result of opposing forces acting on the organisation and on individuals. He described these forces as driving and restraining forces producing a 'quasi stationary equilibrium'. The opposing pressures of driving and restraining forces produce a temporary state of balance. In order to promote the right conditions for change, to understand what is happening and to understand the forces of resistance to change, Lewin recommended the technique of force field analysis. The restraining forces should be identified with a view to removal, and then the driving forces would push forward to again achieve the quasi stationary equilibrium previously described. Refreezing would happen in the final stage. Again, even if the theory does not produce the change, analysing the forces aids understanding and subsequent communication. Figure 12.4 shows an example of a force field analysis in midwifery; it can be helpfully used as part of the diagnosis phase.

A simple chart that lists the driving and restraining forces of a particular change can help midwives see the problem more clearly and can help to focus their energies in the right direction. Too often teams become so trapped in the intricacies of off-duty rotas and on-call lists that they lose sight of the original aim. Sometimes it can be just one individual whose particular views or idiosyncrasies are preventing change. This analysis can help in the diagnosis and analysis of resistance.

Soft system methodology

The task ahead is neither easy nor straightforward. It must be planned, carefully considered and evaluated. Soft systems methodology is one of the most useful methods of evaluating organisational change. According to Checkland (1991), the approach allows the organisation to redefine systems as the programme develops. In the light of the complexities associated with implementing 'Changing Childbirth' the evaluation and review of the proposed system of care is essential. Soft systems methodology requires a conceptual model of the whole system involved in the change. Sometimes the drawing of a 'rich picture' to describe aspects of the change and see where the change is can be really helpful, especially if

Figure 12.4   *Force field analysis*

ACTUAL: Fragmented maternity services

OPTIMAL: Continuity of carer for all women during the childbirth
              experience

PROBLEM: Traditional ways of organising care are still the norm

GOAL: For women to have improved satisfaction with the childbirth
              experience

Driving forces for change ⟶	*Restraining forces* ⟵
Consumer demand, pressure groups, etc.	There is nothing wrong with the present system
The market economy and a growing awareness of customer rights	Mortality and morbidity rates are improving
Formal and informal leaders, e.g. writers, lay organisations	Thought by some midwives to represent a minority
Social policy, e.g. 'Changing Childbirth', the John Major 'Charters'	Thought to express the wishes of the middle class minority
Financial. NHS Trusts are self-managing and are obliged to manage their resources effectively and efficiently	Fear of more work, more responsibility for less pay. Deteriorating working conditions and employment rights
Midwives keen to develop their skills	Some are not
Midwives want to raise their professional status and achieve greater autonomy	Some want to opt for a quiet life
Integrated services are more effective in meeting women's needs	Clinical directorates sometimes favour separate departments as being more manageable
Doctors trust midwives with normal birth	Some don't
There is duplication of effort and resources, especially in the community and in GP practices	GPs may lose out financially if they are not involved in maternity care
UK Government statements on the Health of the Nation	Things are OK as they are
World Health Organization goals of 'Health for All'	Does not apply to this area
Birth is not an illness	Labour is only normal in retrospect
Women want a positive experience of childbirth	Women want a normal healthy baby

individual midwives are allowed to contribute their version of events to the picture. The definition of the system tends to change as the work proceeds, and as more and more members of the organisation become involved in the process, the less the resistance that can be expected. Checkland believes that constant review is essential in any change process and believes that failure is more often associated with inadequate diagnosis and review than major strategic errors. He believes that it is crucial not to dismiss apparently trivial concerns but to listen carefully to the detail of concerns.

More about leaders and visions

Burns (1978), writing in support of leaders and change agents in effective change, suggests that organisational change is best led by transformational leaders as opposed to transactional leaders. The transformational leader tends to adopt a strategic vision, leads by sharing the vision and has a longer-term focus. Peters and Waterman (1982) describe the role of the chief executives in successful companies as transformational leaders. They are able to create a culture of participation, energy, change and closeness to the 'customer' through a 'hands on' involvement in the management of the organisation.

The change management 'guru' Kanter (1983), mentioned above, argues that although vision is generally thought to be the task of leaders, people at all organisational levels have a role in bringing about the change that she describes as being part of 'post entrepreneurial life'. She suggests that success is created by a three-part mix: the context set at the top, the values and goals emanating from top management by channels designed in the middle to support those values and goals, and finally project ideas bubbling up from below. She sees leadership operating at all levels rather than just at the level of top management.

Individuals resist change for a variety of reasons, the main one probably being fear. Various theories suggest ways of dealing with resistance by analysing and understanding it. However, many planned changes fail because the wrong strategy has been chosen to implement the change.

Trade unions and others

Traditionally, the role of trade unions has been to oppose and challenge management. They existed to protect the interests of the workforce rather than to support the implementation of change, but trade unions and professional organisations such as the Royal College of Midwives (RCM) do have a role to play in helping midwives to adjust to change and overcome resistance. For many years, the RCM seemed to be pulling in two directions. The professional officers were, for example, responding to the government's agenda and giving evidence to the Health Committee set up to consider the maternity services. They argued in favour of providing women with choice, control and continuity of carer (House of Commons Health Committee 1992). They supported the proposal of improving care for women and advised that care be reorganised in order to provide greater continuity of carer. In supporting and promoting these proposals, they also believed that a reorganised maternity service would lead to an improvement in the status, position and autonomy of the midwife. However, at the same time, the industrial relations department was crying 'foul' when midwives were being asked to change their well-established working practices. The situation has improved with reorganisation (another change!), and now all officers have a professional and industrial relations role. The RCM is first and foremost a membership organisation for midwives. It continues to fight for the rights of its members, in the belief that midwives who are enjoying good working conditions and employment rights will give good care. In her 1995 end of year message, General Secretary Julia Allison said, '1995 has certainly been a year when our trade union profile has been raised significantly'. Her message addresses issues such as pay, clinical grading and professional development but says nothing about women or the need for midwives to change the ways in which they offer care. The needs of midwives, rather than the needs of childbearing women, are now the priority of the RCM.

The role of trade unions has changed significantly in the past decade, the changes in legislation introduced by the Thatcher government having significantly reduced their power and influence. In the 1990s, trade unions have a role in working with organisations and management. Their techniques now include listening, communicating, collaborating rather than confronting, facilitating, negotiating and supporting while continuing to protect the rights and interests of the workforce as they change the ways in which they work.

Selecting the right strategy

The modern language of management has changed from directing, organising and controlling towards flexibility, decentralisation, empowerment, leadership, collaboration and change. The 'new' management led by Peters and Waterman (1982), Kanter (1983, 1989), Peters and Austin (1985), Peters (1987) and others places great emphasis on appropriate interpersonal skills and on valuing individuals and their contribution to the organisation. The choice of strategy depends to a great extent on the beliefs that managers hold about the people they manage, on the speed with which the change must be brought about and on the anticipated efforts of those involved. The anticipated degree of resistance to the change is another variable to be considered.

Bennis *et al.* (1976) identify three predominant change strategies: rational–empirical, power–coercive, and normative–re-educative. Each of these strategies is based on managers' assumptions about what makes individuals and organisations willing to change or resist change.

The rational–empirical strategy is based on the belief that all human beings are reasonable and intelligent, and will select options that offer optimum benefits to themselves and the group. It assumes that knowledge is a major source of power and that, if those who have knowledge and power share this with those they manage, they will understand the reasons behind the change and thus be willing to change. Thus the change is achieved by sharing information and appealing to individuals' logical, rational understanding of the problem.

The power–coercive strategy is based on a different type of power. This strategy is based on the use or abuse of political, legal and economic sanctions to force individuals to adopt the proposed change. The assumption is that the powerless will always obey the powerful or else lose their jobs, lose money, status or privileges. It also makes assumptions about the so-called powerless. Even the powerless have considerable power to thwart the efforts of a manager if the proposals are deemed to be unrealistic, impractical and of no benefit to the employee. These two approaches can be seen as 'shower' or top-down approaches, that is, imposed from top management above.

A third approach is defined as normative–re-educative and assumes that individuals have rights and that people need to be involved in all aspects of the change process. It assumes that change is more likely to be effective and successful if it is owned by those involved. If the proposed change comes from the workforce itself (bottom-up or 'bidet'!), it is even more likely to be supported. The normative–re-educative approach needs open channels of communication and participative management styles. The identification of need for change comes from those who are most closely involved in providing the service and are therefore likely to have the most relevant solutions. It assumes that employees are committed and interested in the job and are keen to progress, develop and change.

Bennis *et al.* (1976) have defined the leadership styles that fit with each of the strategies. In power–coercive strategies, the leader must be directive, tell people what to do, order, instruct and control. In the rational–empirical strategy, the leader has to persuade, sell, enthuse, bargain and convince the employees of the need to change. In the normative–re-educative strategy, the change agent or leader has to negotiate, participate and support with information and advice. The group will be self-directing and will find the solutions to the difficulties and problems that they have identified, but change will not happen quickly.

Kotter and Schlesinger (1988) see the strategic options available to managers as existing on a continuum. At one end, the strategy calls for a rapid implementation, a clear plan of action and little involvement of others; here resistance is merely overturned. At the other end of the continuum, the strategy calls for a slower change process, a less clear plan offering greater flexibility and greater involvement of many more people than the manager or change initiators. They argue that where speed is essential, where the initiators are very powerful, the approach is more likely to involve coercion and manipulation. Where there is a lack of information, where speed is of less importance and where the involvement of the workforce is essential, an approach that includes education and communication is more likely to be effective, albeit slower.

The changes and targets set out in 'Changing Childbirth' and other strategy documents require a major change in the philosophy and organisation of the maternity services. Such changes are likely to need a very time-consuming approach to change that involves participation, involvement, facilitation, support and negotiation. Quick-fix solutions to be implemented next week are doomed to failure.

SUMMARY

From the evidence of this chapter, it is clear that there are no easy answers. Change is painful and difficult to achieve, but midwifery has to change, and many of the rigid, dogmatic practices of the past have no place in the provision of modern health care. It is clear why childbirth has to change; it is also clear that the pressures for change come from many sources. Government policy is easy to see and blame for the disruption, but the pace of technological developments, demographic changes, social change and geographical and world events all contribute to an age of uncertainty.

Theories and models of change help midwives to analyse and understand what is happening, but, as Wilson (1992) warns, the problem in merging theory and application is that many of the assumptions, biases and contradictions of these theories are lost in the haste to apply them. The analysis stage cannot be rushed, and standard answers are not available. The key is to understand the context and thus be able to predict the opposition and the likely outcome of action taken. Other models, such as those described by Marris (1986), help managers to understand the effects of change and deal with the workforce with compassion and sensitivity. The model offered by Rogers (1962) helps in understanding how a group responds to change and helps managers to respect those who are reluctant to go along with change at the beginning. Leaders have a major role in supporting and guiding in a change process. Their skill is in keeping alive the vision of how things might be. They need to be powerful communicators with well-developed interpersonal skills. They need to be able to listen to the laggards and not dismiss their concerns. They need energy, enthusiasm and the commitment of those who share their beliefs and philosophy.

Those whose task it is to manage change need to understand change, the processes and why change is resisted. They need to understand the culture of the organisation and the beliefs and values of those who are employed there. They also need to evaluate and review the process of change at frequent intervals. Those who initiate and manage change have to listen, involve others in the process and be prepared to modify their own cherished ideas and schemes. Many changes fail because of poor interpersonal skills or because managers have selected an inappropriate strategy for change. Strategies frequently reflect the assumptions held about the workforce. It is worth managers thinking about how they would describe the staff of their department to an alien from another planet! If the manager believes in the staff, she or he is more likely to trust them with the task of making the change happen.

There has never been a more important time for leaders in midwifery; managers and leaders, who are not necessarily the same people, need to understand the processes, complexity and nature of change in order to steer the profession through this age of uncertainty.

REFERENCES

Allison J 1995 General Secretary's End of Year Message. *Midwives* **109**(1296):382

Atkinson J 1984 Manpower strategies for flexible organisations. *Personnel Management* **26**:23–7

Atkinson PE 1990 *Creating Culture Change: The key to total quality management.* Bedford: IFS

Basil DC, Cook CW 1974 *The Management of Change.* London: McGraw Hill

Bennis WG, Benne KD, Chin R, Corey KE 1976 *The Planning of Change.* London: Holt Rinehart & Winston

Brown A 1992 Organisational culture: the key to effective leadership and organisational development. *Leadership and Organisational Development Journal* **13**(2):3–6

Bryar R M 1995 *Theory for Midwifery Practice.* Basingstoke: Macmillan

Burns JM 1978 *Leadership.* London: Harper & Row

Checkland P 1991 *Systems Thinking, Systems Practice.* Chichester: John Wiley

Deal TE, Kennedy AA 1982 *Corporate Cultures: the rites and rituals of corporate life.* Reading, MA: Addison Wesley

Department of Health 1993 *Changing Childbirth. A Report of the Expert Maternity Group.* London: HMSO

Drucker PF 1990 *Managing the Non Profit Making Organisation: Practices and principles.* Oxford: Butterworth Heinemann

Goodstein LD, Burke WW 1992 Creating successful organisation change. *Organisation Dynamics* **4**(8):5–17

Green JM, Coupland VA, Kitzinger JB 1990 Expectations, experiences and psychological outcomes of childbirth: a prospective study of 825 women. *Births* **17**:15–24

Handy C 1991 *The Age of Unreason*, 2nd edn. London: Business Books

Harvey-Jones J 1989 *Making it Happen: Reflections on leadership.* Glasgow: Fontana Collins

Hodnett ED 1993 Support from caregivers during childbirth. In Enkin MW, Keirse MJNC, Renfrew MJ, Nielson JP (eds) *Pregnancy and Childbirth Module, Cochrane Database of Systematic Reviews.* Review No. 03871, 12 May 1993, Cochrane Updates on Disc, disc issue 2. Oxford: Update software. Also Social and professional support in childbirth. In Enkin MW, Keirse MJNC, Renfrew M, Neilson J (eds) 1995 *A Guide to Effective Care in Pregnancy and Childbirth*, 2nd edn. Oxford: Oxford University Press.

House of Commons Health Committee 1992 *Maternity Services*, vol 1 (*the Winterton Report*). London: HMSO

Isabella LA 1990 Evolving interpretations as change unfolds: how managers construe key organizational events. *Academy of Management Journal* **33**(1):7–41

Johnson G, Scholes K 1989 *Exploring Corporate Strategy. Text and Cases.* London: Prentice Hall

Kanter RM 1983 *The Change Masters: Corporate Entrepreneurs at Work.* New York: Counterpoint

Kanter RM 1989, reprinted 1991 *When Giants Learn to Dance.* London: Routledge

Kirkbridge P 1993 Managing Change. In Stacey R (ed.) *Strategic Thinking and the Management of Change.* London: Kogan Page

Kotter JP and Hesketh JL 1992 *Corporate Culture and Performance.* New York: Free Press

Kotter JP and Schlesinger LA 1988 Choosing Strategies for Change. In Mayon-White B (ed.) *Planning and Managing Change.* London: Paul Chapman

Kubler-Ross E 1984 *On Death and Dying.* London: Tavistock

Lancaster J, Lancaster W (eds) 1982 *The Nurse as a Change Agent.* St Louis: CV Mosby

Leavitt HJ 1964 Applied organisational change in industry. In Cooper WW, Leavitt HJ, Shelly MW (eds) *New Perspectives in Organisational Research.* New York: John Wiley

Leigh A 1988 *Effective Change: Twenty ways to make it happen.* London: Institute of Personnel Management

Lewin K 1951 *Field Theory in Social Science.* New York: Harper & Row

Lorsch JW 1986 Managing culture: the invisible barrier to strategic change. *California Management Review* **XXVIII**(2):95–109

Machiavelli N 1513 *The Prince* . (Reprinted by Penguin, Harmondsworth, 1970)

Marris P 1986 *Loss and Change.* London: Routledge & Kegan Paul

Mead D, Bryar R 1992 An analysis of the changes involved in the introduction of the nursing process and primary nursing using a theoretical framework of loss and attachment. *Journal of Clinical Nursing* **1**(2): 95–9

Nadler DA, Tushman ML 1989 Organisational frame bending principles for managing reorientation. *Academy of Management Executive* **111**(3): 194–204

Oakley A, Rajan L, Grant A 1990 Social support and pregnancy outcome. *British Journal of Obstetrics and Gynaecology* **997**:155–62

Ouchi WG 1981 *Theory Z: How American business can meet the Japanese challenge*. Reading, MA: Addison-Wesley

Peters T 1987 *Thriving on Chaos*. London: Pan

Peters T, Austin N 1985 *A Passion for Excellence: The leadership difference*. London: Guild Press

Peters TJ, Waterman RH 1982 *In Search of Excellence: Lessons from America's best run companies*. New York: Harper & Row

Phillips JR 1983 Enhancing the effectiveness of organisational change management. *Human Resource Management* **22**(1/2):183–99

Plant R 1987 *Making Change and Making it Stick*. London: Fontana Press

Rogers EM 1962 *Diffusion of innovations*. New York: Free Press. In Wright SG 1989 *Changing Nursing Practice*. London: Edward Arnold

Sandall J 1995 Choice, continuity and control: changing midwifery, towards a sociological perspective. *Midwifery* **11**(4): 201–9

Schein EH 1986 *Organisational Culture and Leadership*. San Francisco: Jossey-Bass

Wille E 1992 *Quality: Achieving excellence*. London: BCA Century Business

Wilson DC 1992 *A Strategy for Change. Concepts and Controversies in the Management of Change*. London: Routledge

Page numbers in **bold type** refer to figures; those in *italic* refer to tables.